Springer

Milan
Berlin
Heidelberg
New York
Barcelona
Hong Kong
London
Paris
Singapore
Tokyo

G. Garlaschi • E. Silvestri • L. Satragno • M.A. Cimmino

The Rheumatoid Hand
Diagnostic Imaging

Forewords by H.K. Genant and G. Cittadini

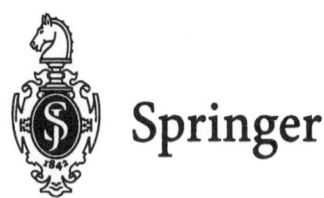

Springer

GIACOMO GARLASCHI
Department of Experimental Medicine
University of Genoa, Italy

ENZO SILVESTRI
Department of Experimental Medicine
University of Genoa, Italy

LUIGI SATRAGNO
MRI Division
Esaote Group
Genoa, Italy

MARCO AMEDEO CIMMINO
Department of Internal Medicine
Division of Rheumatology
University of Genoa, Italy

Contributors

CATERINA AVANZINO
SILVANA D'AVANZO
GIAN MARCO DAZZI
STEFANO DELUCCHI
MARCO FALCHI
FRANCESCO FERROZZI
ALESSANDRA GALLO
ERNESTO LA PAGLIA
SONIA MIGLIORINI

Springer-Verlag Italia
a member of BertelsmannSpringer Science+Business Media GmbH

© Springer-Verlag Italia, Milano 2002
Softcover reprint of the hardcover 1st edition 2002

ISBN 978-88-470-2268-3   ISBN 978-88-470-2266-9 (eBook)
DOI 10.1007/978-88-470-2266-9

Library of Congress Cataloging-in-Publication Data: applied for

Typesetting: Compostudio (Cernusco sul Naviglio, Milano)

Cover design: Simona Colombo

SPIN: 10859469

Foreword

by H.K. Genant

Rheumatoid arthritis (RA) is a systemic disorder of unknown etiology character-ized by articular inflammation and destruction, leading to substantial disability and morbidity. Most patients exhibit a chronic fluctuating course of disease that, if un-treated, results in progressive joint destruction, deformity, disability and even death. It is the most common form of inflammatory arthritis worldwide, with an es-timated prevalence of about 1% and an annual incidence of over 50 per 100,000 women and 20 per 100,000 men in western countries. It frequently affects patients in their most productive years and disability thus results in considerable economic loss. There is no cure for RA, nor means of preventing the disorder, and proper management requires early diagnosis and prompt use of therapies, especially the disease-modifying antirheumatic drugs (DMARDs), to reduce the likelihood of ir-reversible joint destruction.

This volume, *The Rheumatoid Hand*, focuses on important issues, emphasizing diagnosis, management and, especially, magnetic resonance imaging (MRI) at the most relevant site of involvement in RA, namely, the hand. Four authors, repre-senting a multidisciplinary approach, have combined their considerable expertise, along with that of other colleagues, in bringing the readers a depth of experience in clinical diagnosis and management and in medical imaging in patients with RA. The chapters on diagnostic imaging and the galleries of illustrative cases are par-ticularly timely given the recent advances in effective intervention and the requisite for early and reliable diagnosis, as well as for accurate monitoring of these newer therapies. The most powerful and innovative of the medical imaging modalities now available for this task is MRI, because it provides an evaluation of the entire afflicted joint, i.e., the "whole organ assessment." This remarkable technology is the only imaging modality capable of directly visualizing all the components of the joint, including the articular cartilage and synovium, the ligaments, tendons and capsules and, furthermore, of delineating the nature and extent of the gross patho-logic processes evolving in RA. Conventional whole-body MRI has already been shown to be highly reliable in accessing the ravages of this disorder not only in the hand but in most of the other regions affected by RA. A principal deterrent to its widespread use in RA, however, has been limited accessibility and high cost. Now, with the relatively recent introduction of the specialized dedicated extremity MRI system, the potential exists for more universal utilization of a system with lower in-trinsic costs, smaller space requirements, easier installation and greater patient ac-ceptance. Whether broader applications of the dedicated extremity MRI system in screening and monitoring of RA patients will eventuate awaits further knowledge and experience. This volume lends considerable insight into this possibility.

Harry K. Genant, M.D.
Chief, Musculoskeletal Radiology
University of California
San Francisco, CA, USA

Foreword

by G. Cittadini

In certain ways a scientific text can be compared to a literary one. Both spring from the author's awareness and his desire to conceive something meaningful that is worthy of being expressed.

Certainly, in both fields what is considered "meaningful and worthy of being expressed" derives from experiences of different depth, involving precious moments in one's life. However, although in literature that "something" can sail the seas of fantasy, superficiality, and fortuitousness, in science there is no room (I dare say maliciously: "science should not make room") for work that does not divulge something really new or, likewise, is unable to reveal experiences worth revealing.

I suppose we should admit that the authors – two radiologists at the Department of Diagnostic Imaging, San Martino University Hospital, a rheumatologist who has carried out important studies on the prevalence of rheumatoid arthritis (RA) in Italy and Europe, and a technology expert who has played a relevant role in the development of dedicated magnetic resonance (MR) systems – have deposited rich soil on the classic theme "The Rheumatoid Hand". Surely, this soil would bear much fruit if the reader were to venture crossing it in the way the authors themselves have suggested.

Why specifically "The Rheumatoid Hand"? Because, nowadays, the hand is the part of the body most frequently and prematurely affected by joint pain that increases in this chronic, autoimmune, inflammatory disease of the joints, the etiology of which is still unknown, and in which the pathogenesis is the result of multiple factors acting against the background of genetic predisposition.

Why such emphasis on diagnostic imaging? Because, as the authors say, imaging techniques are crucial in the diagnosis, staging, and follow-up of RA patients. If in the past, conventional radiological diagnosis did not recognize the factors shifting the clinical diagnosis arthritis to one of rheumatoid arthritis until it was too late as a result of poor information on cartilage, tendons and soft tissues, nowadays, new imaging techniques, in particular ultrasound and MRI combined, make it possible to bridge the chronic gap: the imaging diagnosis and the diagnosis based on rheumatoid factor research (whose specificity for RA is anything but proven) could be performed almost simultaneously. Their capacity for detecting synovitis, tendon disease, and bone erosions, and also demonstrating synovial pannus hyperemia and quantitating the flow peripheral resistance all play a role in this.

One might ask why there is no approach in terms of nuclear medicine? Because, coherently, the authors wish to present only personal experiences and concerns. Anything that does not involve direct experience is not mentioned, even though inserting a mere bibliographic summary would not have been difficult. Moreover, although the role of radioisotopic diagnostics and radioisotopic synovectomy is now under study at our University Hospital, at the moment, it is too soon to anticipate anything significant.

This semiologic and diagnostic imaging experience is summarized in the presentation of 25 cases, depicting clearly the impact of imaging techniques from a diagnostic and prognostic point of view.

In my opinion, this book, small in dimensions but large in content, will be especially useful to residents in radiology and to radiologists and rheumatologists who are willing to raise their experience and common practice from the first floor, that of conventional radiography, to a higher level, that of the combined study of ultrasound and magnetic resonance.

As is any human endeavor, this book is not perfect (otherwise no foreword would be necessary!) but it is concrete. An example? When the authors say: "even if the exact interpretation of a certain radiographic image resolves, at least in part, a particular diagnostic problem, it is not possible to reach a definite diagnosis without being aware of the patient's clinical condition and without the help of a precise clinical-radiological correlation".

Giorgio Cittadini
Director and Chairman
Department of Diagnostic Imaging
San Martino University Hospital
Genoa, Italy

Contents

1   History, Epidemiology and Clinical Evaluation of Rheumatoid Arthritis

1.1   Introduction

Rheumatoid arthritis (RA) is a chronic, autoimmune, inflammatory disease of the joints that affects subjects of all ages, with a predilection for women of post-menopausal age. Although the etiology of RA is still unknown, its pathogenesis is the result of multiple factors acting against the background of genetic predisposition. Inflammation is probably triggered by nonspecific and as yet unknown infectious agents. The course of RA is usually chronic with alternating periods of exacerbation and abatement. RA is not necessarily confined to the joints but can cause extraarticular manifestations that are frequently severe and sometimes life-threatening.

The history of RA is much debated. The current opinion is that RA is a recent disease, since its first convincing description was published in 1800. The name "rheumatoid arthritis" was coined by Garrod in 1859. However, there are some data deriving from ancient paintings, nonmedical literature and paleopathological studies suggesting that RA could be older than commonly believed.

The classification criteria for RA in current use were developed by the former American Rheumatism Association (ARA), now the American College of Rheumatology (ACR). These criteria are reported in Table 1. They were not developed for diagnostic purposes, but are a useful reminder for the clinician of the characteristics of the disease.

1.2   Epidemiology

The incidence of RA, that is, the number of new cases per year, has been recently evaluated in three studies. In the USA, RA incidence among women participating in a health maintenance program in Seattle was 0.24/1000. In the UK, the annual incidence derived from the Norfolk Arthritis Register was 0.36/1000 in women and 0.14/1000 in men. Finally, a recent study in Finland found an incidence of 0.32/1000. RA incidence becomes higher with increasing age, but in British women this has been confirmed only up to 75 years of age.

RA prevalence, that is, the total number of cases in a defined population, has been the object of many studies. In Caucasian populations from industrialized countries, RA prevalence is between 0.3% and 1.5%. In contrast, RA seems to be rare in Africa and in other developing countries. According to some authors, RA is becoming less frequent and less severe in comparison with studies dating back to the

1960s. This could be due to a change in the risk factors or to the so-called "birth cohort effect". This mechanism implies that the environmental agent triggering RA has been at work in a given period of the past, influencing people born in that time interval. Ever since, the frequency of RA has been declining.

Notwithstanding the limitations of epidemiological studies, both frequency and severity of RA seem to follow a geographical trend, with a higher prevalence in Northern countries and a lower one in the Mediterranean. The possible causes of these differences include genetics, the distribution of age classes, climate, diet, infections and other environmental factors.

1.3 Clinical Features

Today, the characteristics of RA are well defined by the 1987 ARA criteria (Table 1). RA is a symmetric polyarthritis that often involves at onset the small joints of hands and feet, with resulting deformity and disability. It is more frequent in women than in men, with a 4:1 ratio. Its peak of incidence is commonly reported in the 3rd and 4th decades, but recent data suggest that the peak has shifted to the 5th and 6th decades. A clinical course with early morning stiffness and possible systemic manifestations, such as anemia, fever, and fatigue, is classical (Table 2).

Table 1. ARA 1987 criteria for the classification of RA, traditional format

1. Morning stiffness
2. Arthritis of 3 or more joint areas
3. Arthritis of hand joints
4. Symmetric arthritis
5. Rheumatoid nodules
6. Serum rheumatoid factor
7. Radiographic changes

Table 2. Extraarticular manifestations of RA

Nodules
Anemia
Pleuritis
Interstitial pulmonary fibrosis
Bronchiolitis obliterans organizing pneumonia (BOOP)
Pericarditis
Secondary Sjögren's syndrome
Episcleritis
Peripheral neuropathy
Glomerulonephritis
Amyloidosis
Rheumatoid vasculitis
Felty's syndrome *

*Seropositive, nodular rheumatoid arthritis associated with splenomegaly and leukopenia.

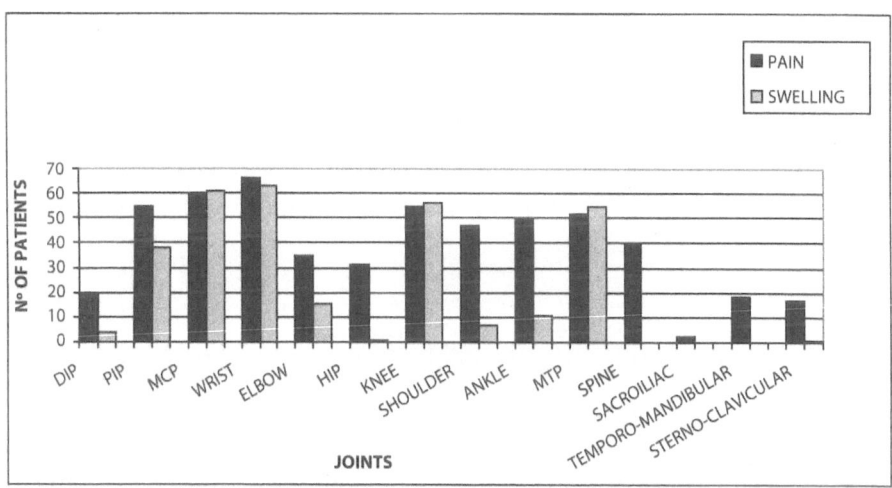

Fig. 1. Localization of joint pain and swelling in 80 consecutive patients with RA

However, RA can also start as a monoarthritis, as a palindromic rheumatism (i.e. intermittent episodes of arthritis with complete remission in between), or with an extraarticular manifestation such as pleuritis. Later on, RA patients can experience spontaneous or treatment-induced remission in about 15-30% of cases, a progressive course in 20%, or a remitting course, with alternating exacerbations and periods of fair control of symptoms, in about 50% of cases.

All diarthrodial joints, which are coated by the synovial membrane, can be involved by RA. The small joints of the hands and feet (proximal interphalangeal joints or PIP, metacarpophalangeal joints or MCP, and metatarsophalangeal joints or MTP), wrist, ankle, shoulder, elbow, hip, and knee are more frequently affected. Figure 1 shows the joints involved by RA in a series of 80 consecutive patients from our unit. The joints affected by RA are swollen because of synovitis and of synovial fluid effusion. They are painful and tender on pressure and passive motion. The most frequently reported symptom of RA is obviously pain, followed by stiffness. However, pain in or around the joints of patients affected by RA is not always due to RA inflammation. Sometimes pain can be caused by mechanical abnormalities of the joint or by associated fibromyalgia. Careful examination of the patient will allow this differential diagnosis in most instances. In late RA, anatomical damage

Table 3. Risk factors for RA progression

Female sex
High titer IgM RF
High number of involved joints
Presence of extraarticular manifestations
High functional disability
Shared RA epitope
Low social class
Poor education

to the joint represented by erosions, ankylosis, luxations, and instability is common. Joint damage due to RA is the combined result of disease activity and disease duration. Therefore, long-lasting RA is almost invariably associated with important structural damage. Risk factors for a progressing course of RA are listed in Table 3. Although RA is commonly considered a disabling but not life-threatening disease, there is compelling evidence that mortality is increased in patients with this disease. Survival of RA patients is similar to that of patients with Hodgkin's lymphoma.

1.4   Evaluation of Patients with Rheumatoid Arthritis

1.4.1   Laboratory Investigations

The acute-phase reactants are most useful for monitoring disease activity and response to treatment. Erythrocyte sedimentation rate (ESR) and C-reactive protein (CRP) are the preferred tests both in the clinical setting and in controlled trials. CRP is well correlated with radiological progression of RA. It is more sensitive to changes of disease activity and less influenced by other noninflammatory conditions, with the exception of infection.

Rheumatoid factors (RFs) are a group of antibodies against the Fc fragment of denatured IgG, which are produced by B lymphocytes of the synovial membrane. They are classified according to the class of the immunoglobulin. IgM RF is usually evaluated in most laboratories and is positive in about 2/3 of RA patients. It is the only laboratory test included among the ACR criteria. IgM RF is not specific for RA, for it occurs in several other diseases such as Sjögren's syndrome, various connective tissue diseases, tuberculosis, and HCV infection. Interestingly, RF can precede the onset of RA by years. In addition, healthy subjects with RF are at increased risk of developing RA.

Some patients with RA are characterized by the presence of antiphospholipid antibodies, antikeratin antibodies or antibodies to perinuclear factor. The former may be associated with a high incidence of thromboembolic events. Antiperinuclear factor antibodies have a high sensitivity and specificity for RA.

1.4.2   Clinical Evaluation

Counting swollen and tender joints is helpful for evaluating disease severity and patients' follow-up. Joint swelling is associated with anatomical damage, whereas tender joint count is more sensible for treatment-related changes.

Measuring disability is an important part of the evaluation of patients with RA. Several instruments have been developed, such as the disease-specific HAQ (Health Assessment Questionnaire) and AIMS (Arthritis Impact Measurement Scale), or the nonspecific SF-36. These instruments can predict RA evolution at least as well as radiography and CRP measurement.

1.4.3 Imaging Techniques

Imaging techniques are crucial in the diagnosis, staging, and follow-up of RA patients. This aspect will be considered in depth in the main part of this book.

1.4.4 Composite Indexes

Combinations of laboratory tests, clinical findings, and imaging have been developed to better evaluate disease activity, improvement, remission, and the patient's response to treatment. Two examples of these indexes are the Van Der Hejde and the CASI.

1.5 Etiopathogenesis

A simple model of the etiopathogenesis of RA, which is similar to those proposed for other autoimmune diseases, includes infection-induced activation of the immune system against as yet unidentified antigens (collagen, virus, superantigen?) in genetically predisposed individuals. The modulation of the immune system by hormonal, reproductive, mechanical, and environmental factors is gradually becoming understood.

The main target of inflammation in RA is the synovial membrane that covers the internal part of the joint capsule, bursae and tendon sheaths (Fig. 2). Typical features of synovial inflammation are lymphocyte migration in follicles, macrophage migration, neoangiogenesis, and mechanical stress of the joint. Rheumatoid synovitis is characterized by an expansion of superficial cells, including macrophages and fibroblast-like cells, that contribute to the formation of the synovial pannus, a locally invasive tissue that erodes cartilage and bone.

A role for genetic predisposition is supported by the increased concordance for RA in monozygotic as compared to dizygotic twins. RA-associated HLA class II molecules include the HLA DRB1 gene, which codifies a specific amino acid sequence called shared RA epitope. The "shared epitope" is similar to sequences of several common organisms, such as the gp120 glycoprotein of Epstein-Barr virus or the "heat shock protein" of different bacteria. RA patients show an increased immune reactivity against these proteins. This allele is important because the unknown antigen that can trigger RA interacts with the groove produced by the HLA molecule on the surface of macrophages. Recognition of this antigen by the host immune system after macrophage presentation is the primary event in RA. DRB1*04 (DR4) alleles are associated with RA, at least in the Anglo-Saxon population, and are a risk factor for severe disease. In the Mediterranean population, the association between RA and DR4 is less significant. Recent Italian data suggest that DR4 is not associated with RA, extraarticular manifestations, or IgM RF seropositivity. However, Italian patients with HLA DRβ1*04 alleles have more erosions and a higher radiological damage score.

The onset of RA is probably an antigen-driven event mediated by T lymphocytes. T lymphocytes of the synovial membrane are polyclonal in vivo.

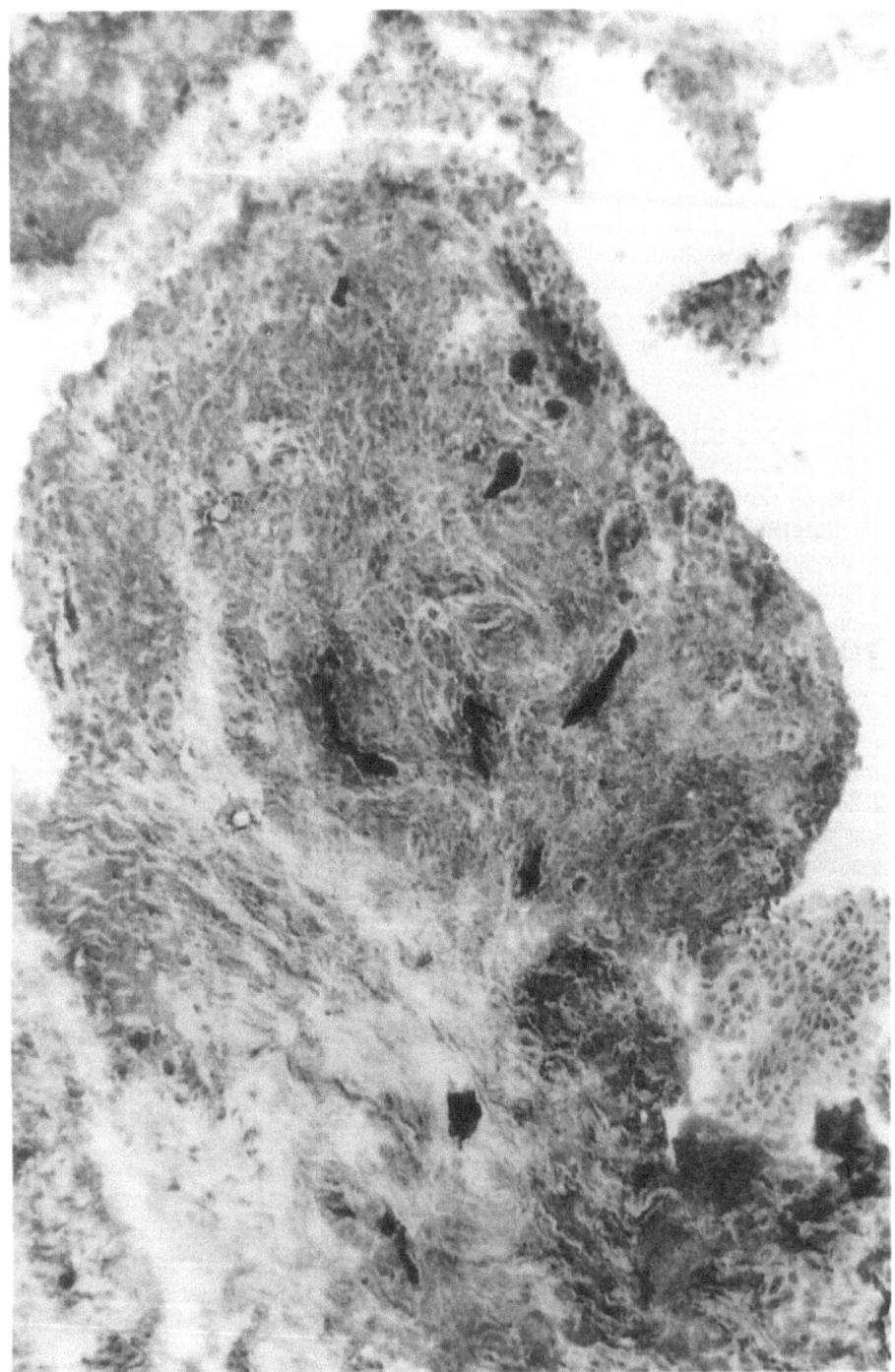

Fig. 2. Typical rheumatoid synovitis with villous formation showing prominent angiogenesis in the inflamed stroma and superficial lining hyperplasia (alkaline phosphatase, hematoxylin counterstaining x 100)

No specific RA- subpopulation has been identified to date, although these T cells belong mainly to the TH1 subtype which produces interferon-γ. There is a subsequent cytokine-mediated involvement of neutrophils, macrophages, B lymphocytes, and memory T lymphocytes that produces high amounts of different cytokines. Angiogenesis is a crucial event in the destructive process caused by synovial pannus. It is elicited by different cell types and their products, such as fibroblast growth factors, vascular endothelial growth factor, and several soluble adhesion molecules which are upregulated by hypoxia and inflammatory cytokines. These cytokines are mainly produced by macrophages and fibroblasts, which regulate the production of metalloproteases, cell proliferation, recruitment of new cells into the joint, and expression of inflammatory mediators. This response is probably the cause of the chronicity of RA synovitis.

1.6 Therapy

Treatment of RA is based on different types of drugs and interventions:
- Nonsteroidal antiinflammatory drugs (NSAIDs)
- Steroids
- Disease-modifying antirheumatic drugs (DMARDs) or disease-controlling antirheumatic therapy (DC-ARTs)
- Biologicals
- Additional therapies (gastroprotection, intraarticular injections, patient education, physical therapy, occupational therapy, surgery....)

NSAIDs are essential for the symptomatic treatment of RA patients. They allow control of pain and stiffness and can be used in every phase of RA. The mechanism of action of NSAIDs is complex. Their main activity is the inhibition of cyclooxygenase, an enzyme that metabolizes the arachidonic acid of membrane phospholipids to prostaglandins. Unfortunately, cyclooxygenase is also involved in the production of prostaglandins, which are important in maintaining renal flow and integrity of the gastrointestinal mucosa. This fact explains the possible side effects of this class of drugs, which include renal insufficiency and peptic ulcer disease. Recently, two types of cyclooxygenase (COX-1 and COX-2) have been identified. Different NSAIDs have a different affinity to these two types. The ideal NSAID should be able to inhibit inflammatory COX-2 but not the protective COX-1. Several new NSAIDs with a favorable profile of COX inhibition have been recently marketed or are in the final stage of development. However, cyclooxygenase inhibition is not the only mechanism of action of NSAIDs.

Steroids are among the most potent antiinflammatory drugs. They can be used at intermediate dosages in the early stages of severe RA for several months, and at reduced dosages thereafter. Doses of 5 mg of prednisone daily are considered to be relatively safe. Possible side effects include weight gain, hypertension, diabetes mellitus, osteoporosis, and increased risk of infections and of peptic ulcer disease, especially if associated with NSAIDs. A possible role of steroids in slowing the progression of radiographically detected damage is still debated.

DMARDs should be used in an early stage of RA, soon after the diagnosis has been confirmed. The concept of disease modification is not accepted by most rheumatologists and the new term of "disease-controlling drug" has therefore been introduced. However, most DMARDs affect process and outcome variables at least in medium-term studies. In mild RA, treatment can be based on sulfasalazine, hydroxychloroquine or a combination thereof. In more severe cases showing risk factors of rapid progression of the disease, methotrexate is the drug of choice, followed by cyclosporin A. Methotrexate is active and well tolerated also in elderly people. In an open study, progression of structural RA damage was shown to be reduced by cyclosporine. Combination therapy is a novel approach to the treatment of resistant RA. The basic concept is that the association between two or more of the above-mentioned drugs will increase their efficacy without the risk of more severe side effects. Different combinations have been proposed, including methotrexate-hydroxychloroquine-sulfasalazine or methotrexate-cyclosporine. This approach should be tailored to the individual patient with careful weighing of benefits and risks. Finally, it should be considered that also in patients with low levels of clinical and laboratory inflammation disease can progress to high degrees of anatomical damage and disability. Therefore, it is recommended to carefully monitor these patients and to treat them appropriately. A new DMARD in clinical use is leflunomide.

The latest advance in the treatment of RA is biologically engineered drugs directed against immune-competent cells or their cytokine products. Two types of anti-TNFα antibodies have been recently marketed in most countries. One is a chimeric IgG monoclonal anti-TNF antibody; the second is a recombinant soluble TNF receptor. They have been proved to be dramatically effective in acute flares of RA inflammation. Recent data suggest that they can reduce radiological progression of RA. Their safety profile is not completely known, and some concern has been raised about the risk that they may reactivate latent infections. In addition, the high cost of these compounds is a matter of discussion. At present, the role of these highly effective drugs in the therapeutic strategy of RA is not completely clear.

2 Diagnostic Imaging

2.1 Conventional Radiography

Conventional radiography has always played a major role in the diagnosis and follow-up of RA. Since 1957, when the ARA published the first classificative criteria of the disease, conventional radiography, together with laboratory and clinical findings, has been included among the required criteria.

In accordance with these criteria, several authors have tried to develop quantitative methods based on "radiographic scores" in order to have a tool for diagnosis and therapeutic follow-up (Table 4). These methods, however, are hampered by the lack of an universally accepted X-ray imaging protocol and the extremely variable inter- and intra-observer measurements.

The need for an earlier diagnosis and the recent technological innovation in diagnostic imaging, such as ultrasound and magnetic resonance, have made conventional radiography a more and more complementary technique in RA evaluation. It has the advantage of being a well-known and established technique but, due to poor information on cartilage, tendons and soft tissues, it applies to a largely irreversible stage of the disease.

Table 4. Common methods based on "radiographic scores": the relevant parameter for each method is indicated (from A. Giovagnoni et al./Eur J Radiol 27, 1998)

Method	Soft tissue edema	Juxtaarticular osteoporosis	Bone erosions	Articular space narrowing	Ankylosis	Sub-luxations
Steinbrocker	-	*	*	*	*	*
Berens	*	*	*	*	*	*
Sharp	-	-	*	*	*	-
Larsen	*	*	*	*	-	-
Genant	-	-	*	*	*	-
Kaye	-	-	*	*	*	*
Rau and Herborn	*	*	*	*	-	-

Even if "digital X-rays" allow manipulation of image contrast and zoom, for a better evaluation of bone and periarticular soft tissues, reducing the number of exposures, the main limitation of this technique still remains.

In order to give a detailed and complete overview of some of the available diagnostic imaging methods in the evaluation of the rheumatoid hand, the capabilities, the limitations and the technical study protocol of conventional radiography will be analyzed in the following section.

2.1.1 Examination Techniques and Normal Radiographic Anatomy

A correct X-ray approach to the study of the rheumatoid hand includes standard views, possibly followed by specific views in order to answer specific clinical questions.

The examination should always be performed using all necessary technical adjustments (fine focus, high-definition screen and films, correct use of diaphragms and exposure time) to have a correct evaluation of the single anatomical structures of the hand and the wrist.

The following is the detailed description of the standard and specific views (Table 5), as usually performed in the study of the rheumatoid hand:

Table 5. Standard and specific views in the study of the rheumatoid hand

Standard views:
- neutral posteroanterior view
- semipronated oblique view
- neutral lateral view

Specific views:
- posteroanterior view in ulnar and radial deviation
- carpal tunnel view
- specific carpal bone views (scaphoid, triquetral)
- specific finger view

2.1.1.1 Standard Views

Neutral Posteroanterior View

The palm is held in the plane of the forearm and flat on the film cassette. The long axis of the third metacarpal and distal radius are parallel. The central ray of the X-ray beam is centered on the cassette and directed through the back of the carpus at the midpoint of the interstyloid line for the evaluation of the wrist and through the midpoint of the third metacarpal bone for the study of the hand (Fig. 3).

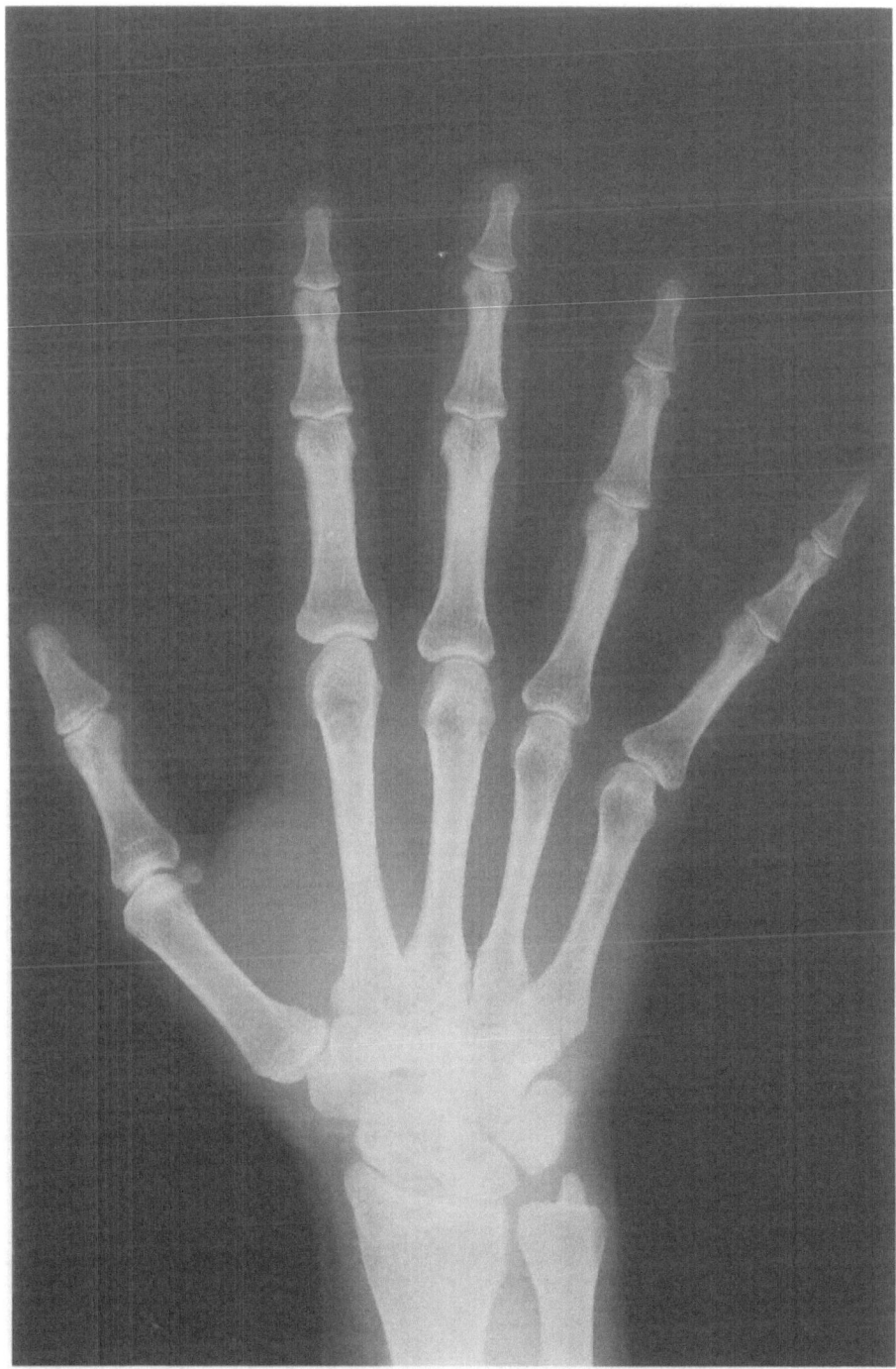

Fig. 3. Neutral posteroanterior view

Semipronated Oblique View

The forearm is held in pronation and the radial side of the hand is slightly elevated; stretched fingers slightly bent, with thumb and forefinger opposed, separated by a radiotransparent spacer, allowing a good evaluation of the examined joints (Fig. 4).

Neutral Lateral View

The forearm is aligned with the wrist, flat on the film cassette on the ulnar side; fingers in extension and thumb adducted. The central ray of the X-ray beam is centered on the scaphoid. This view allows the evaluation of possible volar or dorsal deviation of the wrist (Fig. 5).

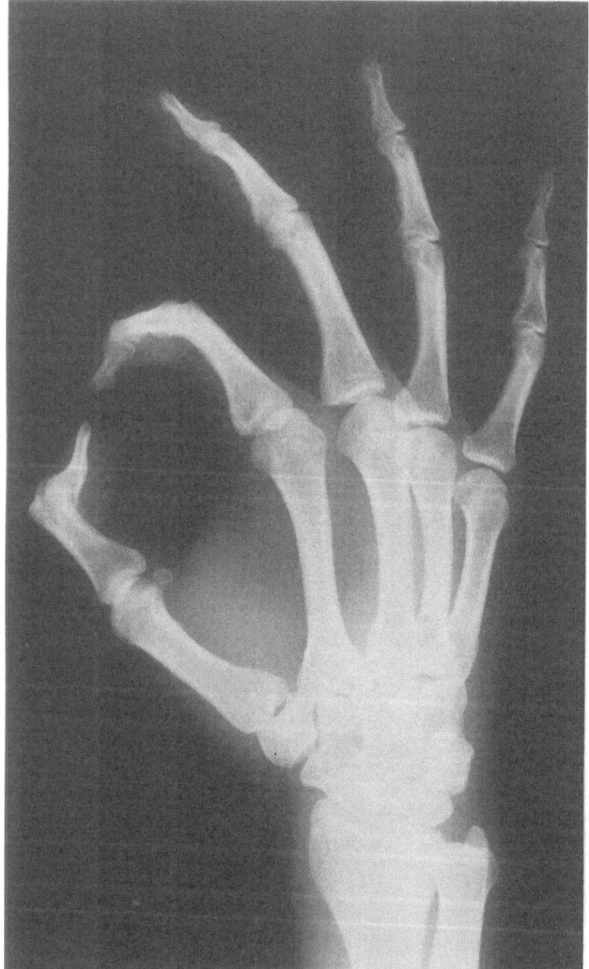
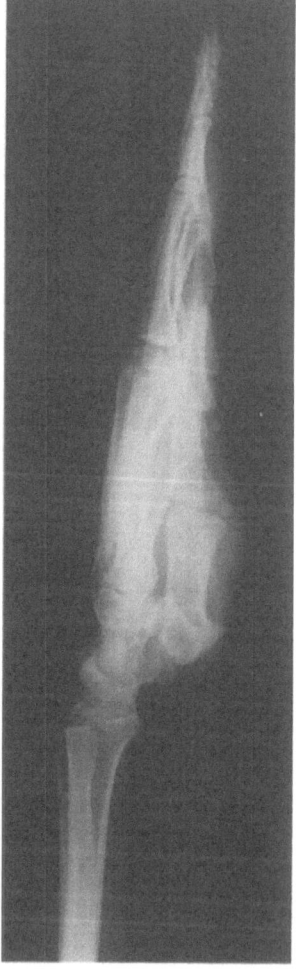

Fig. 4. Semipronated oblique view   **Fig. 5.** Neutral lateral view

2.1.1.2 Specific Views

Dorsopalmar Projection in Ulnar and Radial Deviation

The hand is in maximum ulnar or radial deviation with extended fingers and the palmar surface of the wrist leaning on the X-ray cassette. The central ray of the X-ray beam is centered on the midpoint of the interstyloid line, at the level of the capitate. Both views are extremely useful in the evaluation of the carpus (Figs. 6, 7).

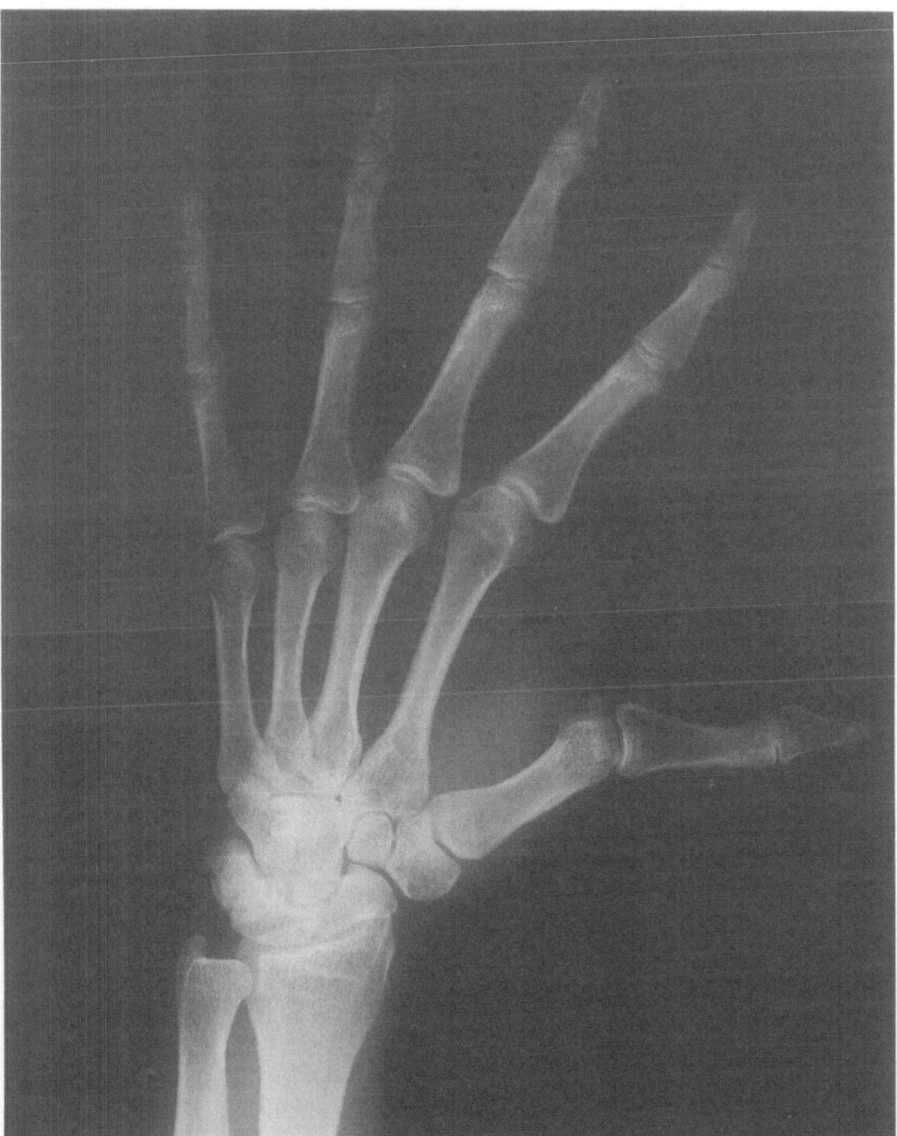

Fig. 6. Posteroanterior view in ulnar deviation

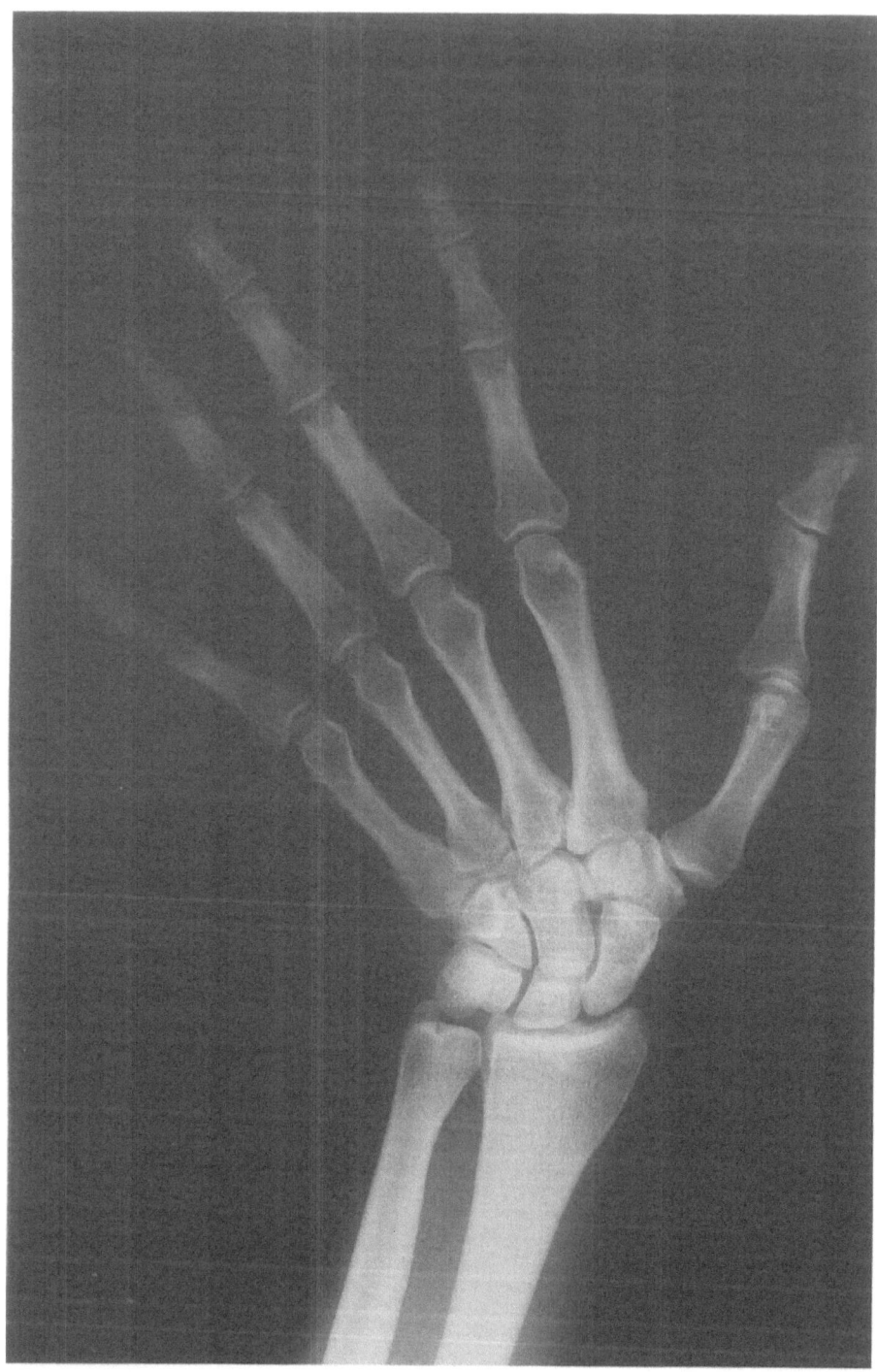

Fig. 7. Posteroanterior view in radial deviation

Carpal Tunnel View

The palm of the wrist is held on the film cassette with the hand in prone position and in dorsal flexion, in order to obtain a perfect 90° angle between the major axis of the hand and the film cassette (this position can be maintained with the help of a band).

The central ray of the X-ray beam is parallel to the carpal tunnel.

This view allows a good demonstration of the hamate and the hook of the hamate, and an evaluation of indirect signs of flexor tendons tenosynovitis (Fig. 8).

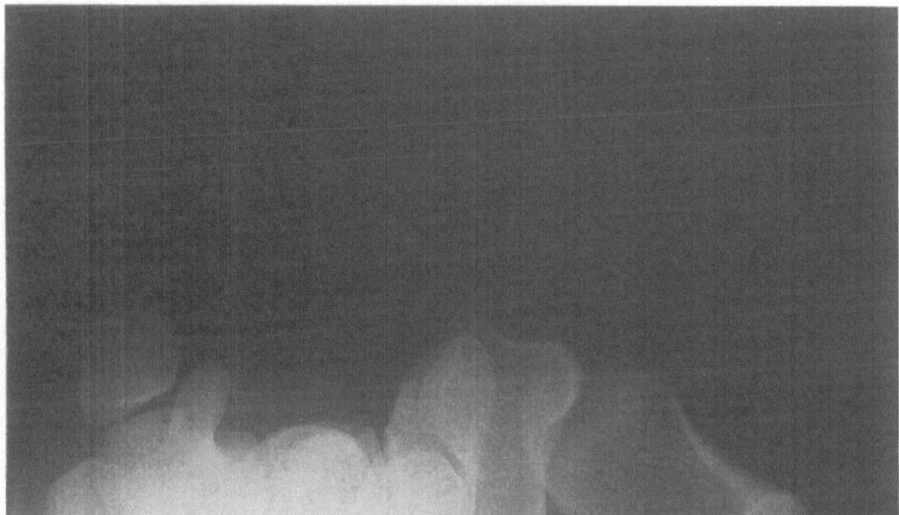

Fig. 8. Carpal tunnel view

Specific Carpal Bone Views (Scaphoid, Triquetral)

The palm of the wrist is held on the X-ray cassette, the hand in ulnar deviation with the thumb aligned with the radius and the other fingers in flexed position. The central ray of the X-ray beam is centered on the third radial of the interstyloid line (Fig. 9).

Specific Finger Views

MCP and IF joints should be examined with orthogonal and oblique views, in order to avoid adjacent joints overlapping (Fig. 10).

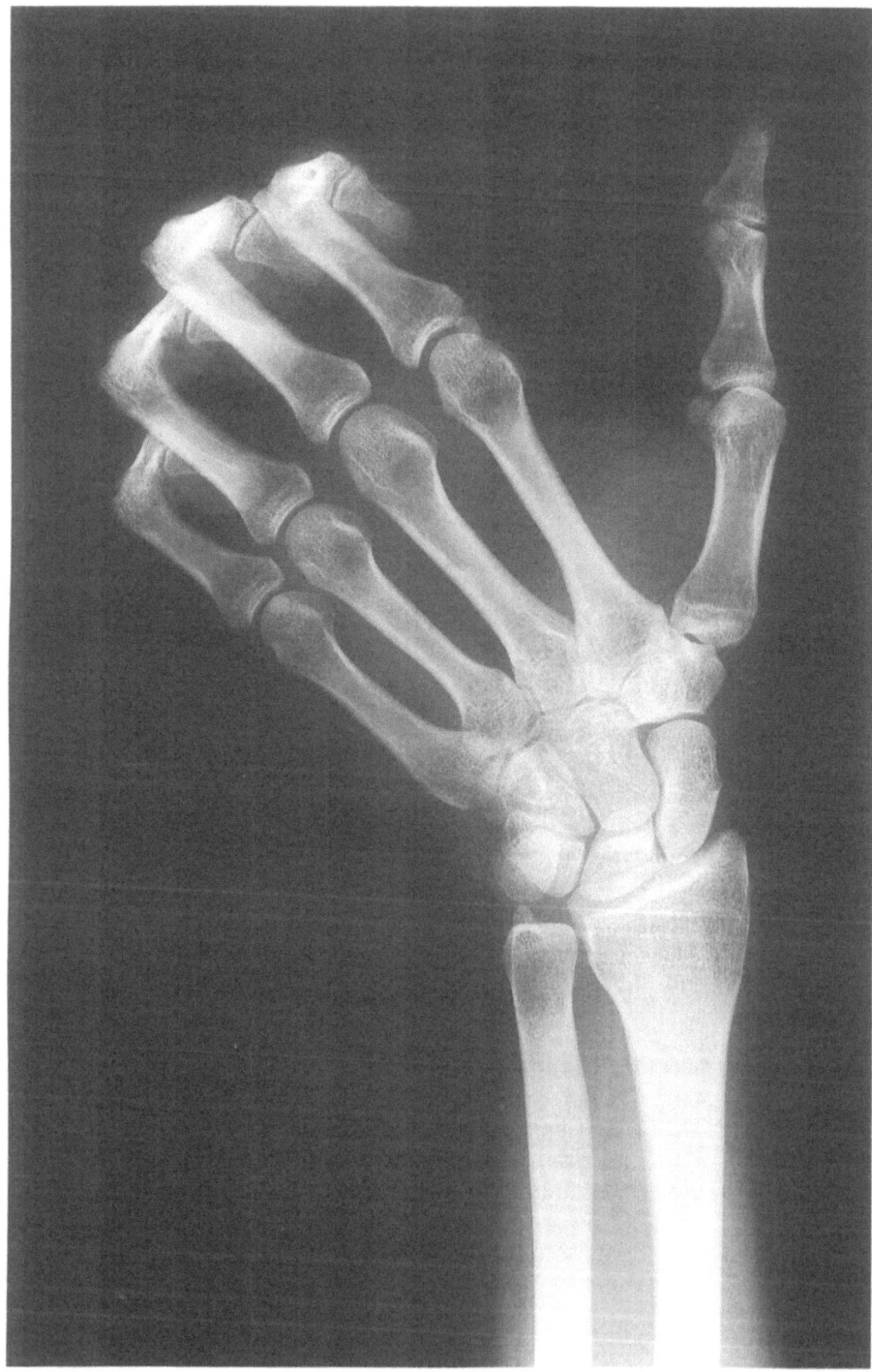

Fig. 9. Scaphoid view

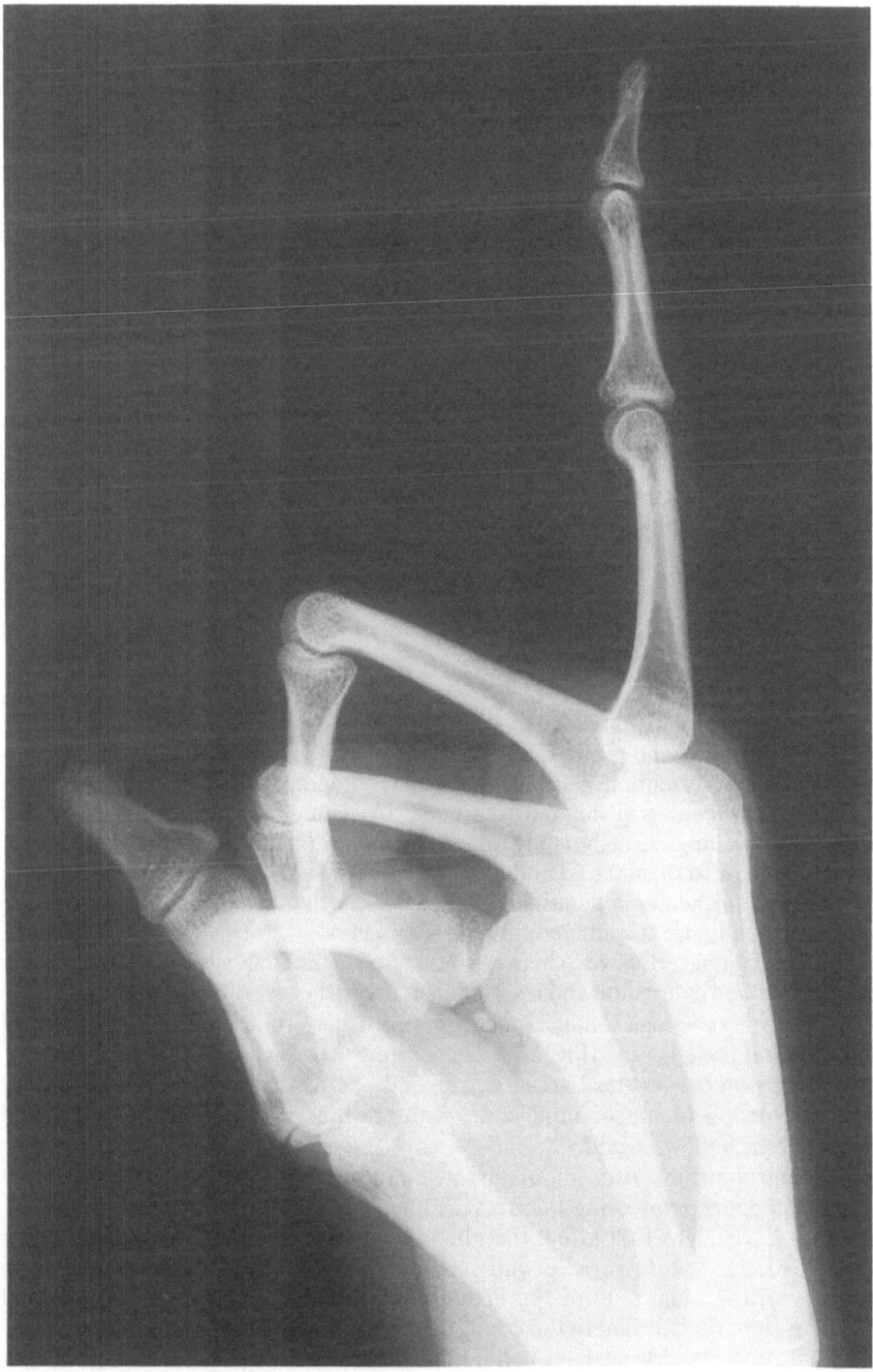

Fig. 10. Lateral view for the study of the second finger

2.1.2 Conventional Radiography and Rheumatoid Arthritis

Synovial membrane hypertrophy, effusion and pannus are the most important findings in the intraarticular phase of RA. Articular cartilage and subchondral bone lesions characterize the intermediate and the advanced stages of the disease, and are mostly secondary to synovial inflammation. In Table 6 radiological findings are correlated to the pathological changes in RA.

Table 6. Pathological-radiological correlations in RA

Pathological changes	Radiological findings
Synovial inflammation and fluid effusion	Soft-tissue edema and joint-space widening
Hyperemia	Osteoporosis
Bare cortical areas destruction	Erosions
Invasion of articular cartilage by pannus	Joint-space narrowing
Subchondral bone destruction	Erosions and subchondral cysts
Involvements of capsule and ligaments	Deformities, subluxations, fractures, fragmentations and sclerosis
Fibrous or ossified tissue formation	Bone ankylosis

Acute synovitis is the first manifestation of the disease, characterized by exudation, cellular infiltration and proliferation, local edema with increase of intraarticular fluid and capsular distension. The corresponding radiographic pattern is characterized by aspecific widening of the joint space and by symmetric (fusiform or eccentric) soft-tissue swelling, corresponding to non-directly distinguishable tendon sheath inflammation, or to rheumatoid nodules.

Capsular thickening may usually be detected in the metacarpal heads as disappearance of adipose subcutaneous tissue (Fig. 11).

The prevailing "effusive" character of acute rheumatoid synovitis, strictly connected to blood congestion and hyperemia, is the first cause of bone alterations. The characteristic radiological appearance is periarticular osteoporosis with thinning of subchondral bone lamina (Fig. 12). As consequence of synovial proliferation, erosive lesions on bare cortical areas, destruction of covering cartilage with exposure and destruction of subchondral bone, with multiple radiotransparent areas and pseudocystic hollows, occur.

Radiographically, after initial narrowing of the joint space, an irregular bone surface appears, expressing the irreversible articular damage caused by inflammation. Early signs first affect the ulnar side of the wrist, appearing as irregularities of the styloid process and secondary involvement of the triquetrum. Moreover, the ulnar side of the distal epiphysis of the radius the radiocarpal compartment (expanding to the contiguous scaphoid bone in its mediolateral aspect not protected by cartilage) and, finally, the distal carpal bones (Fig. 13) are involved.

In the hand, the MCP joints and the PIP joints, particularly of the second and third

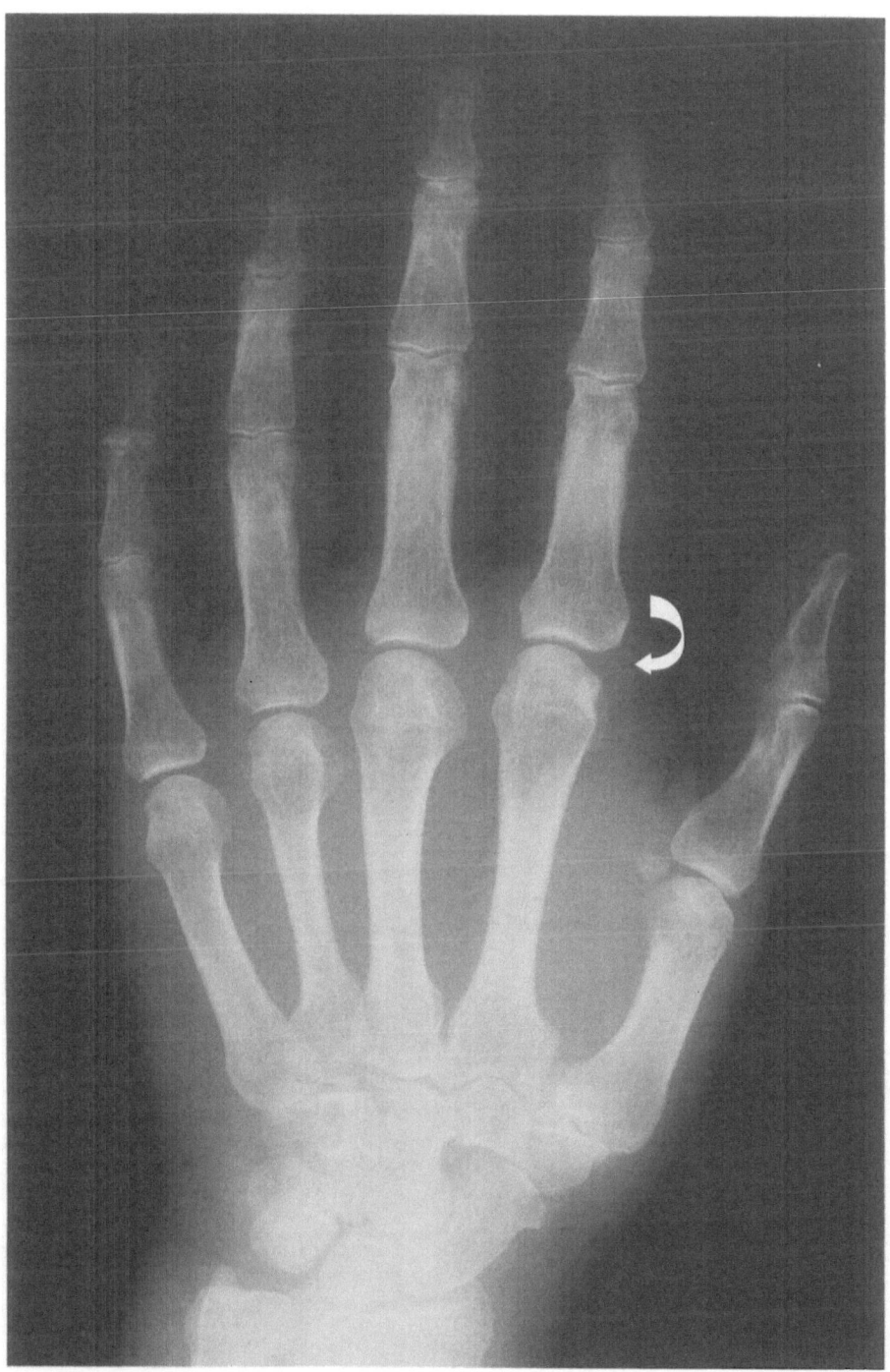

Fig. 11. Posteroanterior view of the wrist. The soft-tissue swelling and the early widening of the joint space (*curved arrow*) are clearly visible

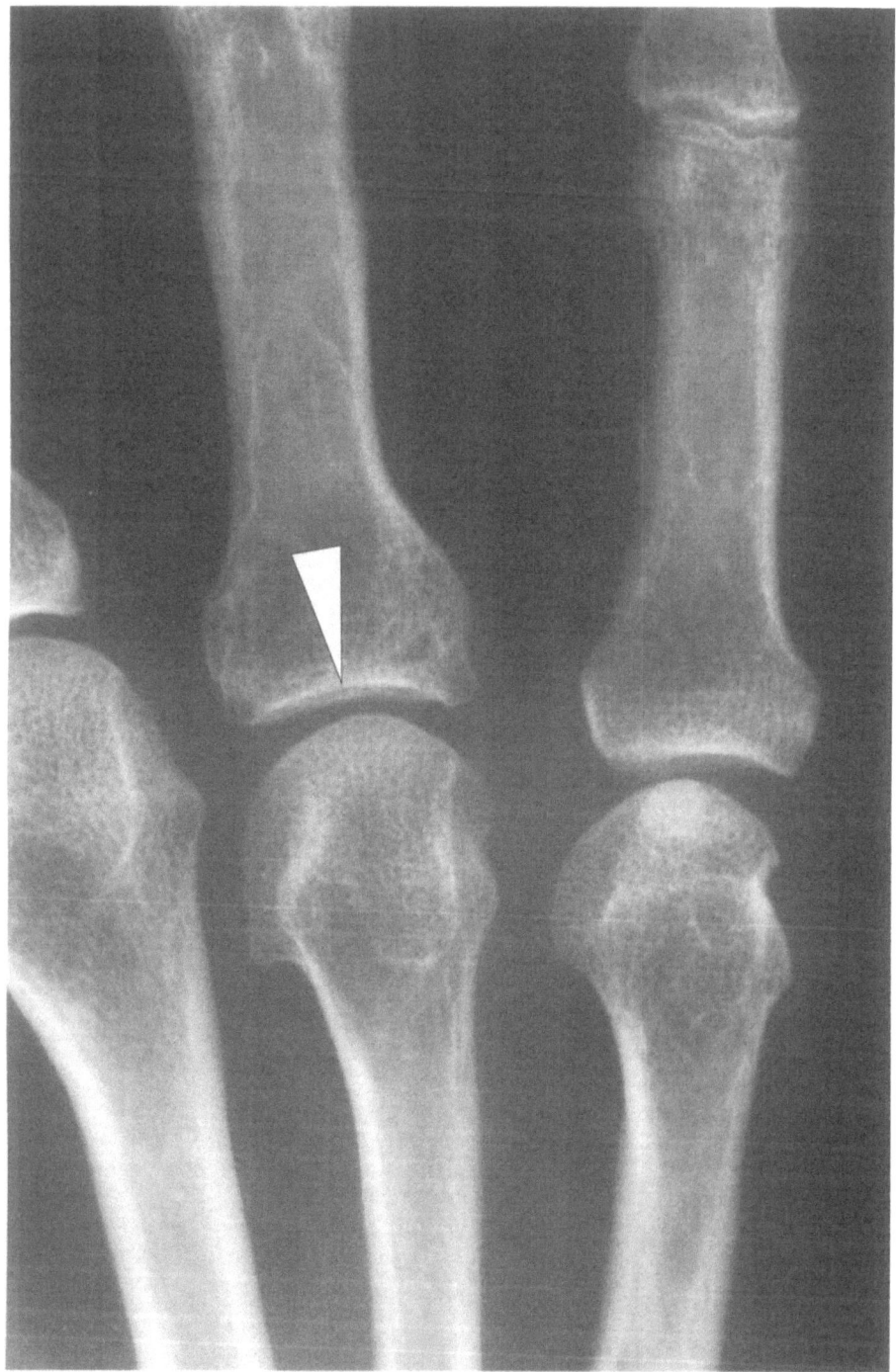

Fig. 12. Posteroanterior view of the MCPs. Early juxtaarticular osteoporosis with mild thinning of the subchondral bone (*arrowhead*)

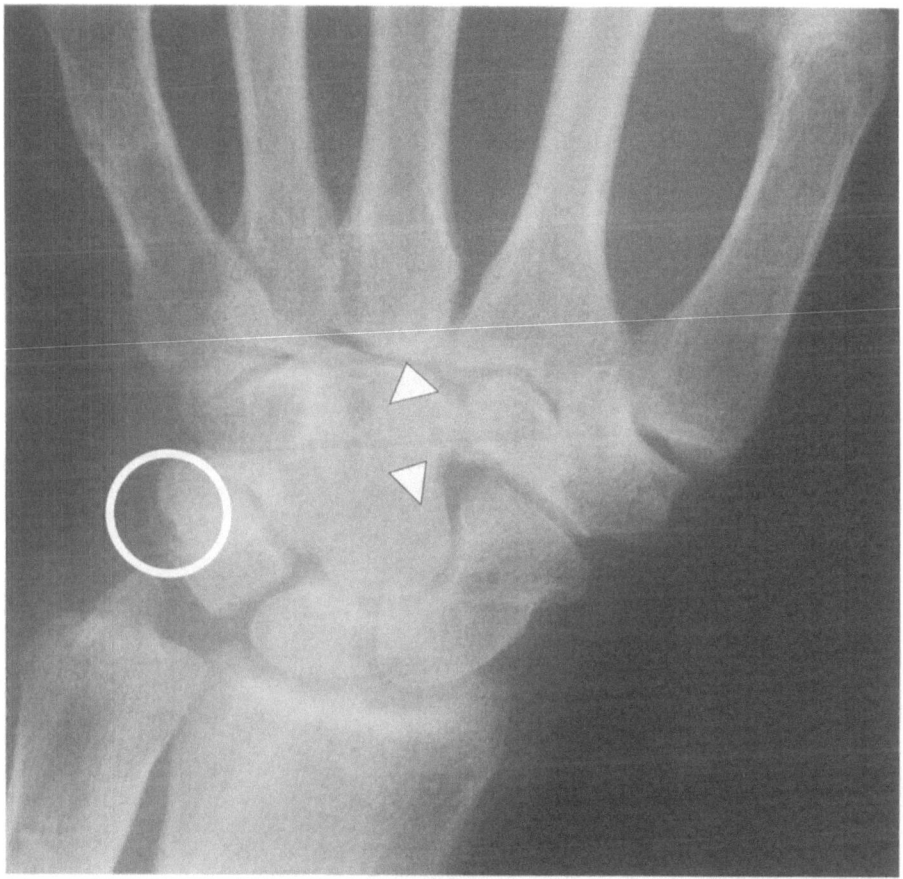

Fig. 13. Posteroanterior view of the wrist. Minimal irregularities of the triquetrum articular surface (*circle*) and subtle cystic alterations of the capitate (*arrowheads*)

fingers, are typically involved. These changes affect more frequently the proximal head, not protected by articular cartilage (Fig. 14).

The distal interphalangeal joints (DIP) may occasionally have marginal erosions, less extended than the proximal ones, and they usually express the superimposition of an osteoarthritic process (Fig. 15).

The persistence of the inflammatory process results in irreversible and highly disabling alterations. The marginal erosive process (Fig. 16) may become severe with deforming structural joint changes associated with tendons and ligaments involvement more evident in the fingers (ulnar deviation and subluxation in MCP joints); irregularity of bone surfaces due to erosive processes may cause an altered alignment of the wrist with medial shift of the proximal carpal series and "ulnar head syndrome", due to dorsal subluxation of the latter and diastasis of the lower radio-ulnar region, caused by destruction of fibrous, cartilaginous and ligamentous supporting structures. All these lesions are best seen in a lateral view.

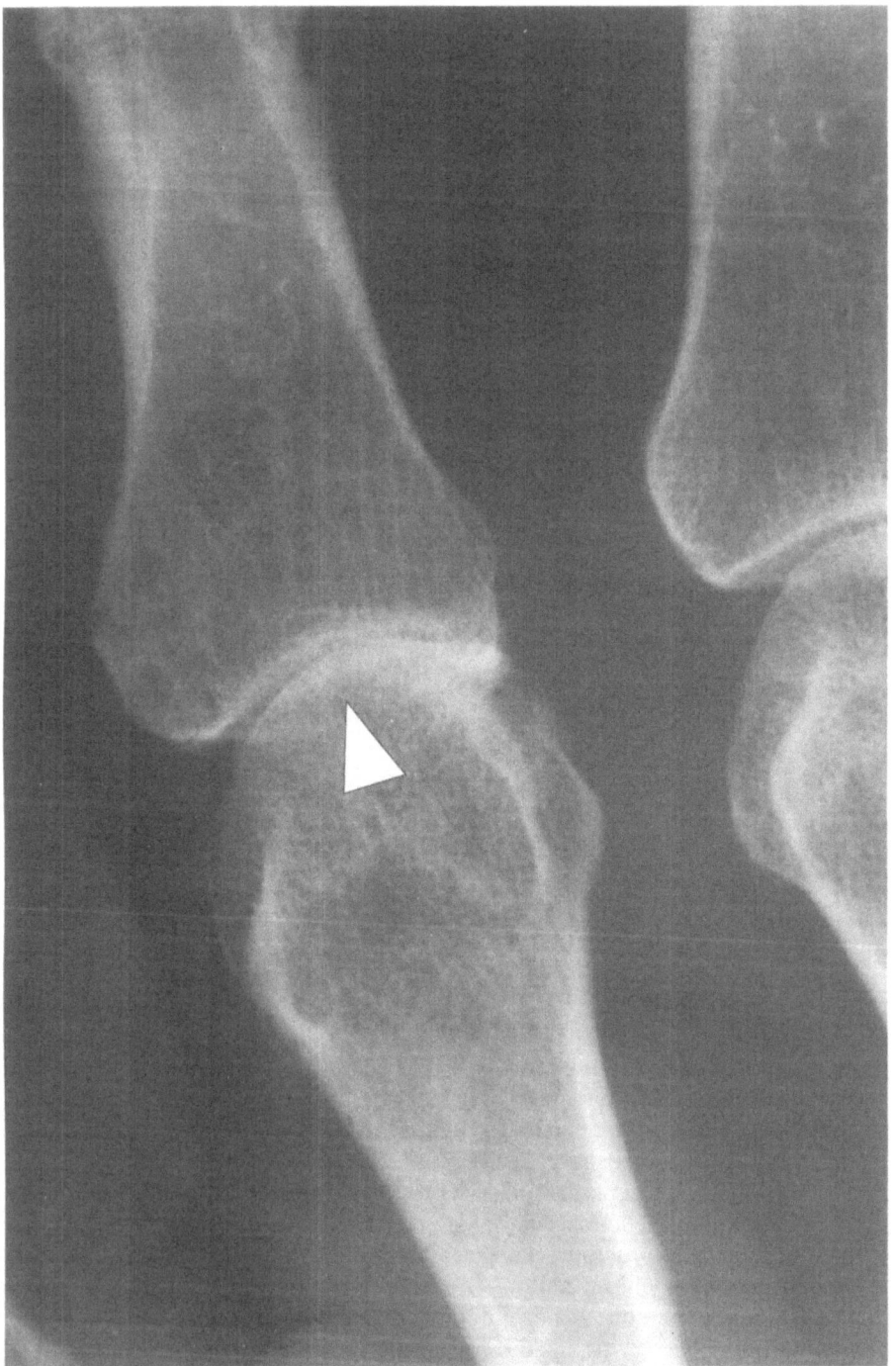

Fig. 14. Posteroanterior view of the hand. Reduction of the second MCP joint space. Minimal cortical irregularities of the second metacarpal head are also demonstrated (*arrowhead*)

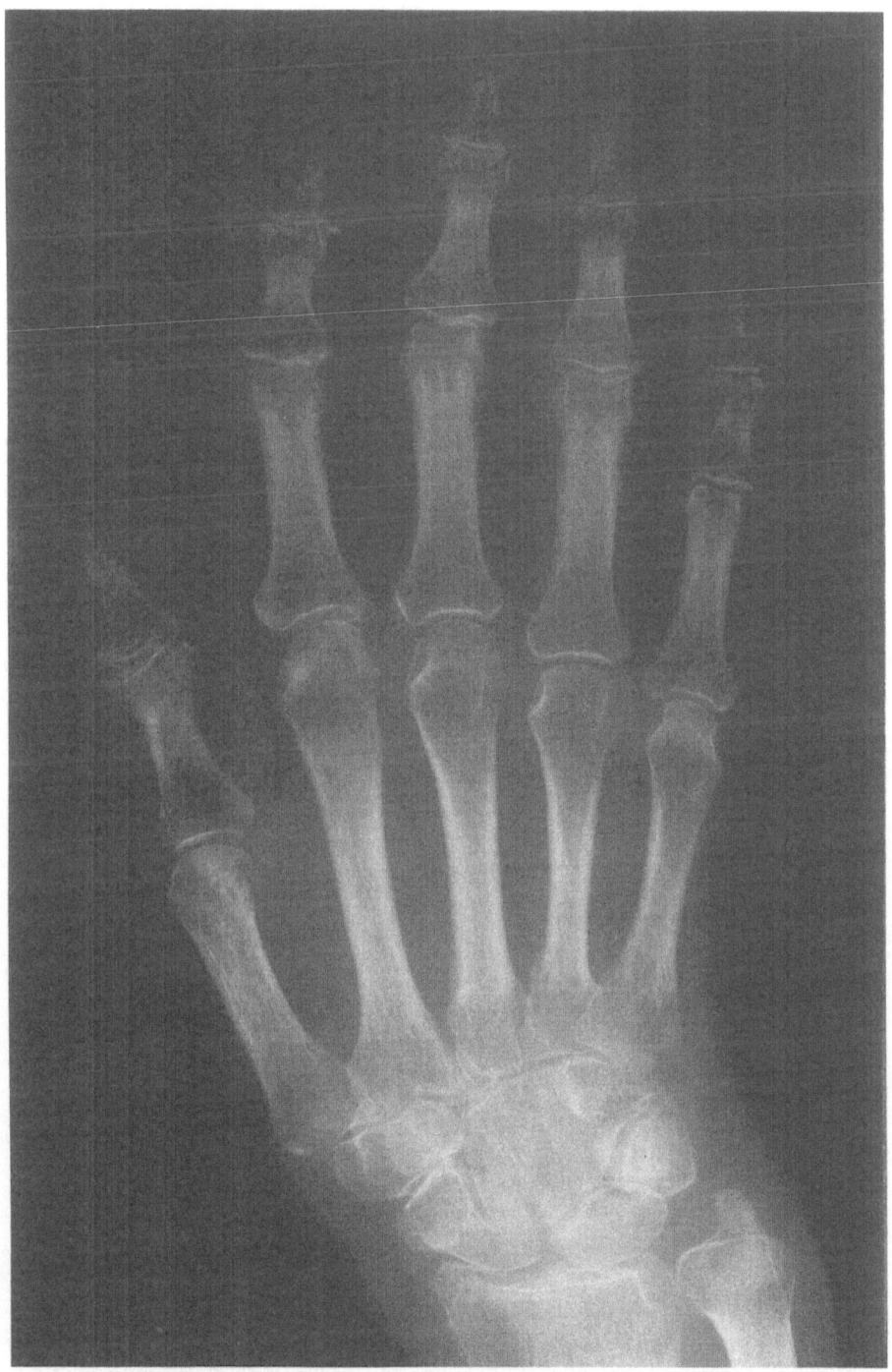

Fig. 15. Posteroanterior view of the wrist. Large erosions are seen in the first metacarpal head and are associated with marked narrowing of the DIP joints due to degenerative osteoarthritis

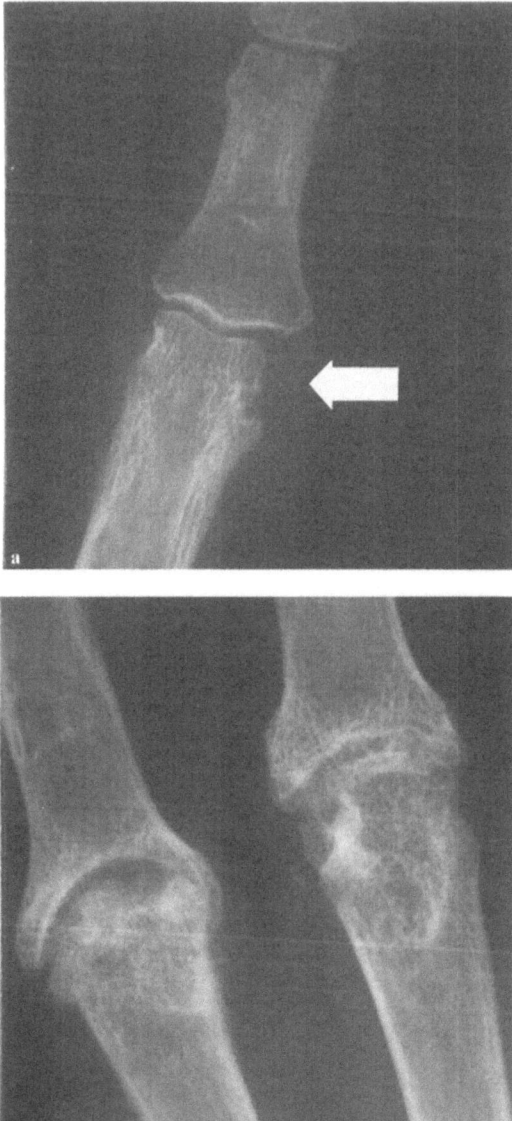

Fig. 16a, b. Posteroanterior views of the hand. **a** Marginal erosion of a proximal phalanx (*arrow*). **b** This view well demonstrates a large erosion at the first MCP joint level

Finally, when carpal synovial involvement includes all structures, a progressive joint space narrowing or even obliteration can occur, with resulting possible fibrous or, more rarely, bony ankylosis, that can be easily demonstrated on X-rays (Figs. 17, 18).

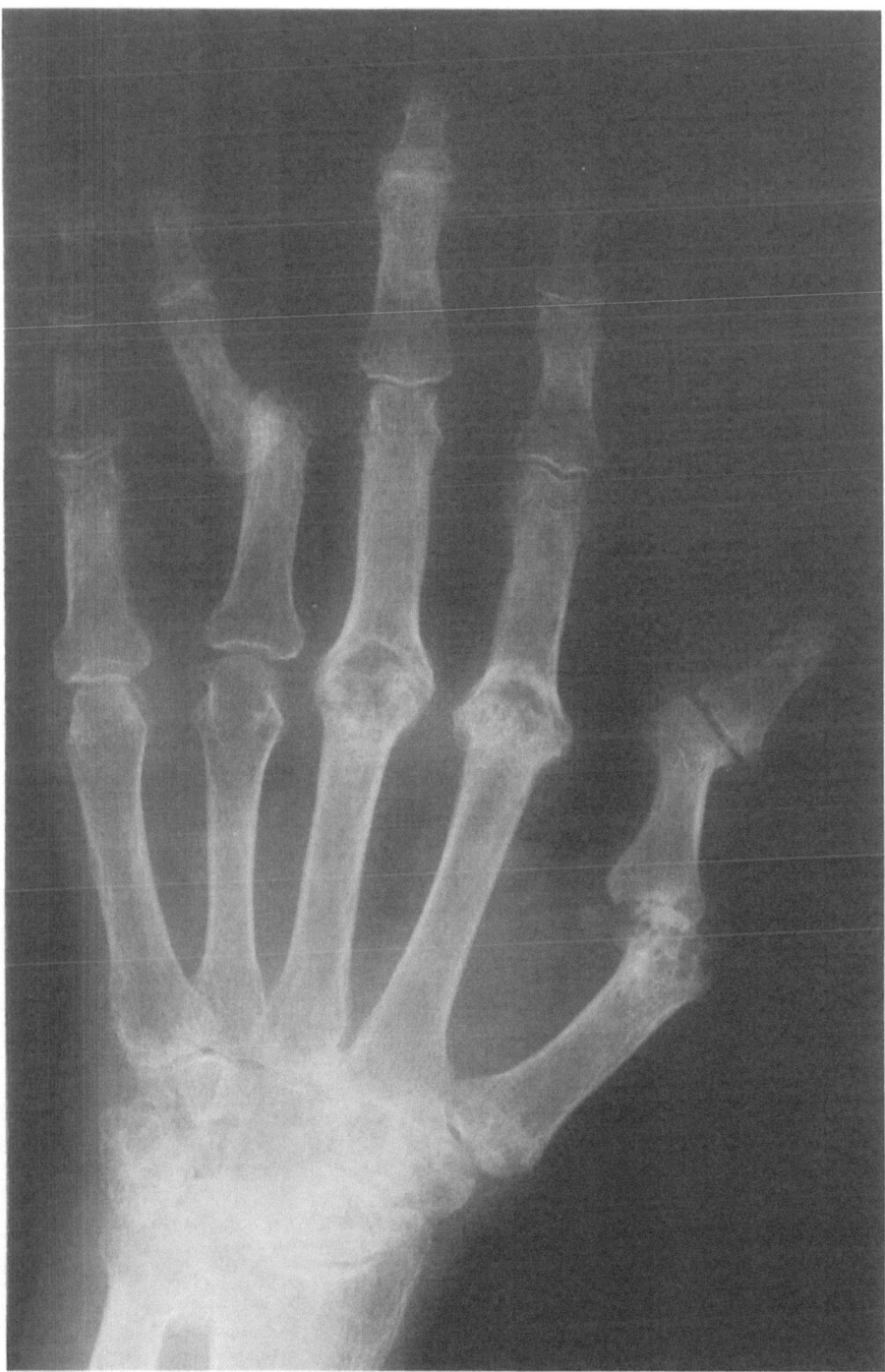

Fig. 17. Posteroanterior view of the wrist. Multiple erosive and pseudocystic lesions typical of RA with signs of subluxation and dislocation of some involved joints

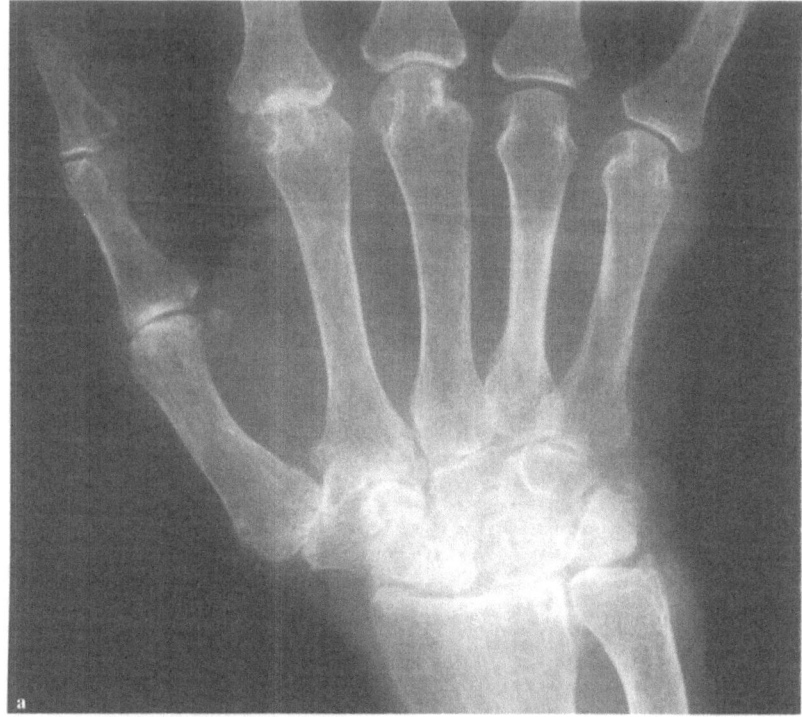

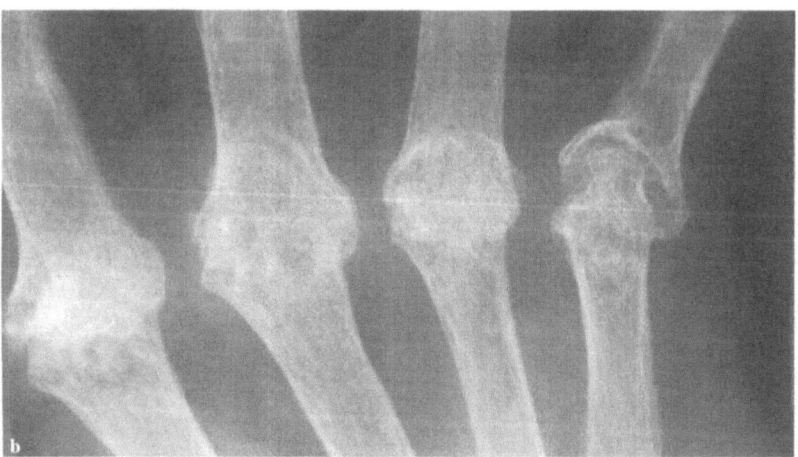

Fig. 18a, b. Posteroanterior view of the wrist. Carpal (**a**) and MCP (**b**) ankylosis

2.2   Ultrasonography

Recent technological innovations, together with the development of high-quality software, the introduction of high-frequency transducers and new Doppler systems, and the use of newly developed contrast agents, have made ultrasound (US) a very helpful technique in the diagnosis of rheumatoid arthritis. By merging the information gained from US with spectral analysis through the Doppler technique it is possible to monitor the state of inflammation according to the level of hyperemia and flow resistance.

2.2.1   Transducers

The US imaging quality is related to its capacity to render examined structures as closely as possible to anatomical reality. The choice of the transducer is therefore essential, and a compromise must be made between spatial resolution and penetration of the US beam. These parameters are, respectively, directly or inversely proportional to the frequency of the US beam. Therefore, it is clear that in the US examination of superficial structures we should use linear transducers with a frequency of 10 MHz, which is very good for visualizing the anatomical detail of the first 6-7 cm of depth and for a comprehensive view of the explored region given by a nonspecific focalization of the superficial tissues and an optimization of spatial and contrast resolution. When examining the hand, this represents the minimum quality standard for a good US analysis. Actually, the "gold standard" is the use of dedicated electronic linear transducers with a large bandwidth (5-13 MHz) that are able to provide high-quality images for the whole explored area. These transducers utilize a sophisticated technology of multiple focalization, which allows a very good representation of the near field of view, good penetration, and excellent contrast resolution. Moreover, in order to avoid artifacts related to poor superficial focalization and, consequently, poor spatial resolution, it is possible not to use spacers, which are otherwise needed in the examination of the superficial tissues. Very high- frequency probes (from 15 MHz to 20 MHz) are also available which provide exceptionally fine anatomical detail and can be used in selected cases as a second level examination; however, due to the poor comprehensive view, these probes cannot be used as a routine procedure.

2.2.2   Doppler Techniques

The color Doppler technique, which is extremely effective in the evaluation of high/medium speed flows, is not as good in enhancing very slow flows which characterize peripheral areas, such as the musculoskeletal system. A new evaluation modality for the Doppler signal (power Doppler) has been recently developed. Unlike color Doppler, this technique does not provide information on flow speed and direction but rather on signal intensity inside the explored vessels. There are two essential advantages: a wider dynamic interval regarding available power for signal representation and a relative independence from the value of the angle of incidence between US beam and flow direction. This results in higher sensitivity in demonstrating slow flows and in a better representation of the course of irregular and tortuous vessels. The Doppler signal contains information about three flow parameters: speed, direction, and number of the red blood cells in the volume sample. The first two represent the information element of the color Doppler image; the third determines the signal amplitude, that is its intensity, and therefore power Doppler can only identify the presence of the flows and not their directions. Nevertheless, the use of power Doppler in the musculoskeletal system is optimal because the limitations of this technique (absence of aliasing, strong sensitivity to motion artifacts, and impossibility of identifying the flow directions) are not relevant in the peripheral areas where flows are quite always slow, there is slight artifact movement, and the information about flow direction is not of particular significance.

2.2.3 Contrast Agents

Current contrast agents are the latest discovery in US imaging, offering some interesting and useful possibilities in the field of rheumatology. They are stabilized gas microbubbles, conceived so as to amplify insufficient Doppler signals originating from poor and slow flows, which are typical in peripheral areas. Nowadays, routine use of these agents does not seem to be indicated due to both the high cost of the products and their limited application field. However, US contrast agents may offer interesting perspectives, particularly in the field of rheumatology, to support not only in the diagnostic but also in the in the therapeutic phase. As a matter of fact, US contrast agents improve the representation of the state of inflammation, similarly to enhanced CT or MR.

2.2.4 Examination Technique

2.2.4.1 Ultrasonography

US examination should be preceded by a correct technical organization of B-mode parameters. Although all US units are provided with specific programs to examine superficial tissues, it is always necessary to use the maximum available dynamic range to have a complete display of the gray scale, to correctly position the focus on the structures of interest and to optimize the control gain to have an even display of the field of view.

US evaluation should be performed with the patient seated in front of the operator with forearm and wrist positioned on a plane surface at adequate height to be in a neutral and comfortable position. All anatomical regions and their structures (subcutaneous layer, tendons, nerves, muscles, joints, articular recesses, and bone surfaces) should be examined. Finally, dynamic examination should not be forgotten in order to estimate mobility and position of tendons related to peripheral nerves. In addition, comparison with the other hand is extremely important to avoid misinterpretation.

2.2.4.2 Color Doppler and Power Doppler

Doppler examination should be performed paying particular attention to press the transducer only slightly onto the skin, in order not to compress the small vessels of

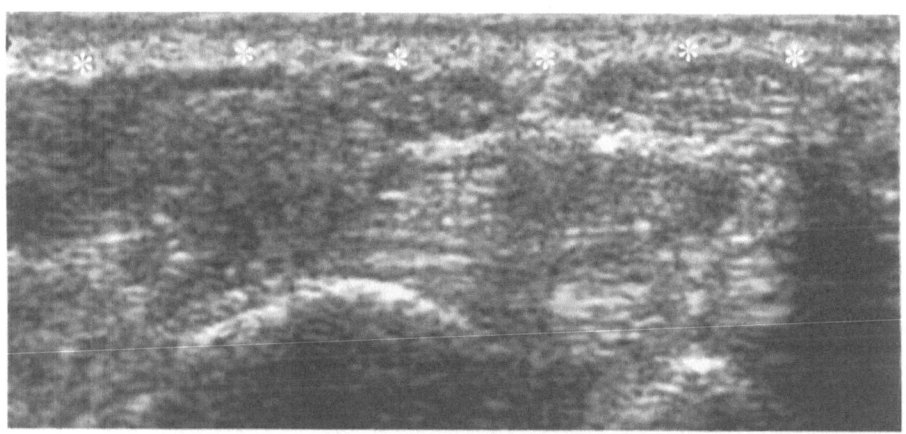

Fig. 19. Transverse scan of the volar aspect of the wrist at carpal tunnel level. The flexor retinaculum appears as a thin hyperechoic band (*asterisks*) covering the flexor tendons and the median nerve

soft tissue on the bones and consequently eliminate the signal. This procedure should be preceded by the best possible setting of technical parameters (low values of PRF*:1000-600 Hz); wall filters (25-50 Hz); gain to maximum possible value allowed by noise; priority filters at 90%; medium-high persistence. The examination should be completed by spectral analysis, to evaluate arterial index. It is possible to use US contrast agents which allow amplification of weak Doppler signals. In this regard we have to remember difficulties due to the *impossibility of estimating signal quantification*, as well as the *absence of standard procedures*. This can be partially compensated by the operator's experience.

2.2.5 Ultrasonographic Anatomy

The US examination of the volar and dorsal aspects of the wrist is performed using transverse and longitudinal scan planes. To avoid possible artifacts due to anisotropy, which could simulate non existing lesions, it is essential to constantly adapt the position of the transducer to the position of the examined structures to assure constant perpendicularity between these and the US beam.

The first structure to be sought along the volar aspect of the wrist is the flexor retinaculum, or transverse carpal ligament, a thin fibrous band covering the carpal tunnel like a roof. The retinaculum inserts itself proximally to the pisiform on the medial side and laterally to the scaphoid, distally on the medial side of the hook of the hamate and laterally to the trapezoid. It is easily recognized on a transverse scan as a thin hyperechoic band having a convex morphology of 3.5-4 mm thickness (Fig. 19).

The superficial and deep flexor tendons of the second to fifth fingers and the longus flexor tendon of the thumb run inside the carpal tunnel. When examined on

* Pulse Repetition Frequency

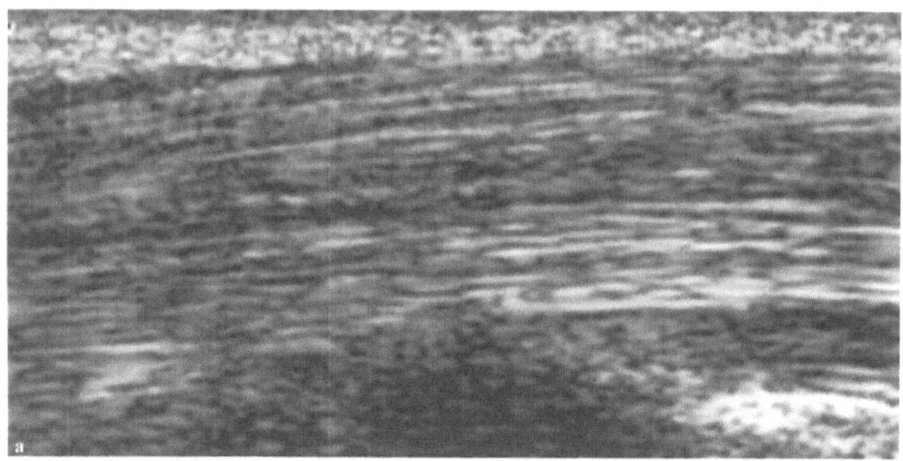

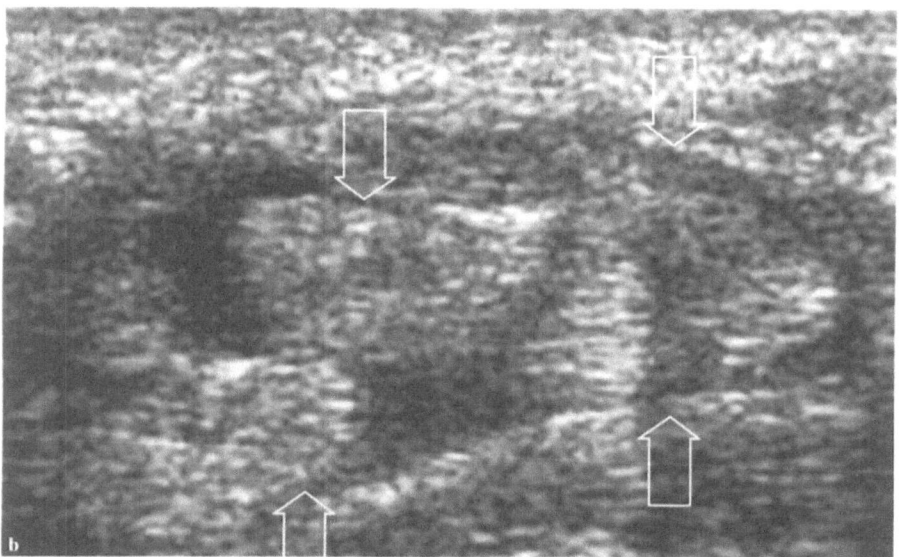

Fig. 20a, b. Longitudinal (**a**) and transverse (**b**) scans of the volar aspect of the wrist at carpal tunnel level. (**a**) The flexor tendons appear as a tubular hyperechoic structure with a fibrillar internal network. (**b**) On a transverse plane, the tendons show the same reflective pattern (*arrows*)

longitudinal planes, these structures look like tubular formations with hyperechoic fibrillar echotexture (Fig. 20a). If they are examined on transverse planes, they acquire a roundish morphology, though maintaining a hyperechoic pattern (Fig. 20b). Transverse and longitudinal scans along the palm of the hand and the fingers allow visualization of their course up to their insertion level. More superficially to the flexor tendons, under the retinaculum, runs the median nerve. It has fascicular echotexture seen longitudinally (Fig. 21a), with ovoid morphology having a larger latero-lateral diameter in transverse scans (Fig. 21b). The median nerve can be easily differentiated from the flexor tendons by four different criteria: site, behav-

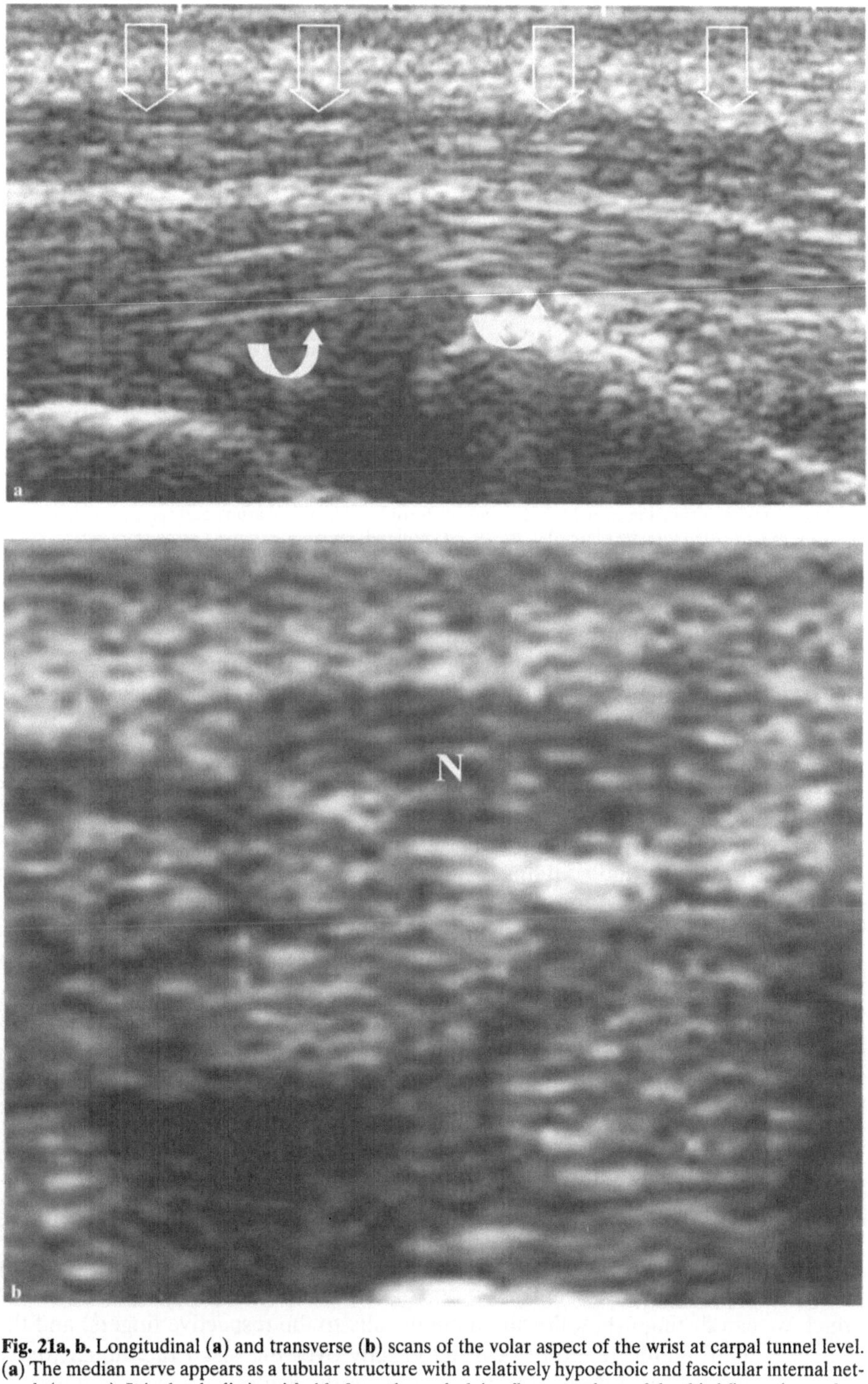

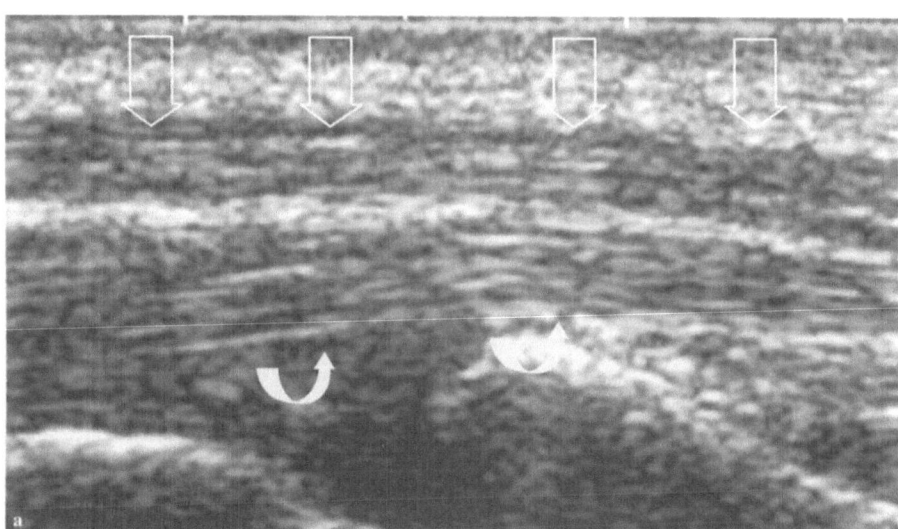

Fig. 21a, b. Longitudinal (**a**) and transverse (**b**) scans of the volar aspect of the wrist at carpal tunnel level. (**a**) The median nerve appears as a tubular structure with a relatively hypoechoic and fascicular internal network (*arrows*). It is clearly distinguishable from the underlying flexor tendons of the third finger (*curved arrows*). (**b**) On a transverse plane, the nerve with the same reflective pattern is clearly demonstrated (*N*)

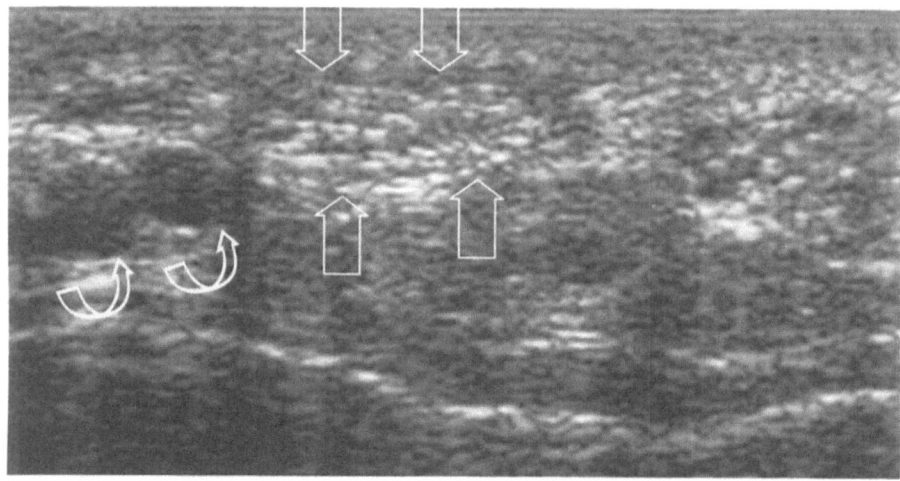

Fig. 22. Transverse scan of the volar aspect of the wrist lateral to the carpal tunnel. The flexor carpi radialis tendon, that runs outside the carpal tunnel, is visible (*arrows*). The radial artery and veins are easily identified as anechoic circular images lateral to the flexor carpi radialis tendon (*curved arrows*)

ior when flexing fingers, echostructure and morphology. The nerve is more superficial than the flexor tendons and does not actively take part in movement during finger flexing, it has a fascicular structure and not a fibrillar one, it is less echogenic than tendons, and, finally, in transverse scans it has an ovoid morphology instead of a roundish one.

Laterally and outside of the carpal tunnel run the tendon of the palmaris longus muscle and the flexor carpi radialis. It is also possible to recognize the radial artery from its anechoic appearance and its pulsatility (Fig. 22).

Medially to the carpal tunnel and laterally to the pisiform bone is the Guyon's canal. It is triangular and contains the ulnar nerve and the ulnar vessels. The ulnar nerve is easily recognized in transverse scan being located medially to the ulnar artery, which appears as a roundish anechoic and pulsing structure (Fig. 23). Proximally to the carpal tunnel, between the flexor tendons and the distal epiphysis of radius and ulna, there is the pronator quadratus muscle. Near the ulnar styloid is the triangular fibrocartilage of the carpus (TFC) (examined on transverse and sagittal-oblique scan planes). It appears like a thin hyperechoic triangle localized just under the extensor *carpi ulnaris* tendon (Fig. 24). The different parts of the TFC complex, i.e., the meniscus, the collateral ulnar ligament, the volar and dorsal radioulnar ligaments, cannot be recognized by US.

In the US examination of the extensor compartment on the dorsal aspect of the wrist, it is most important to locate Lister's tuberculus or the styloid process of the distal radial epiphysis.

In a groove of the colliculus runs the extensor pollicis longus tendon; medially there are respectively, the extensor tendon of extensor digitorum (the single parts of which we can distinguish, following them distally to the respective fingers) and the extensor digiti minimi tendon (localized exactly over the distal radioulnar joint). Clearly visible more centrally, inside a groove in the central surface of the ulna, is the extensor carpi ulnaris tendon (Fig. 25). This tendon can be utilized as an

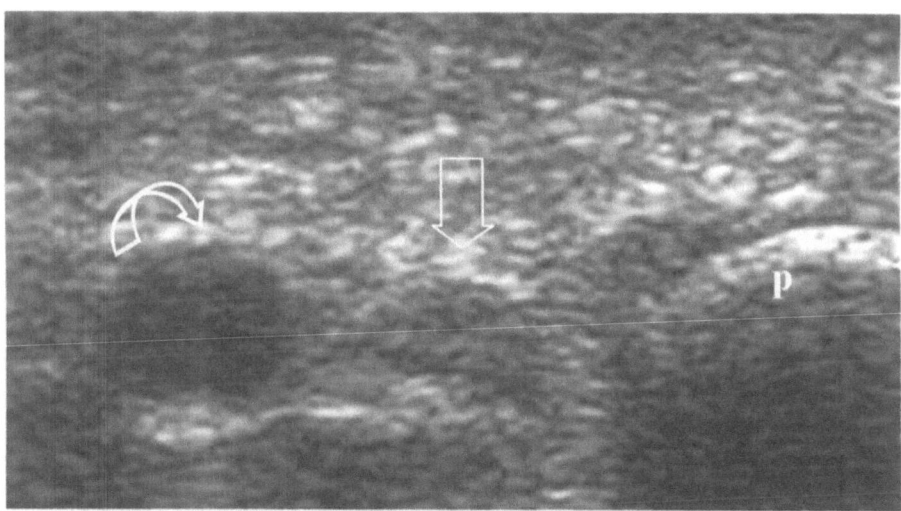

Fig. 23. Transverse scan of the volar aspect of the wrist lateral to the pisiform bone (P). Guyon's canal is visible as a triangular space where the ulnar nerve (*arrow*) and vessels (*curved arrow*) are located

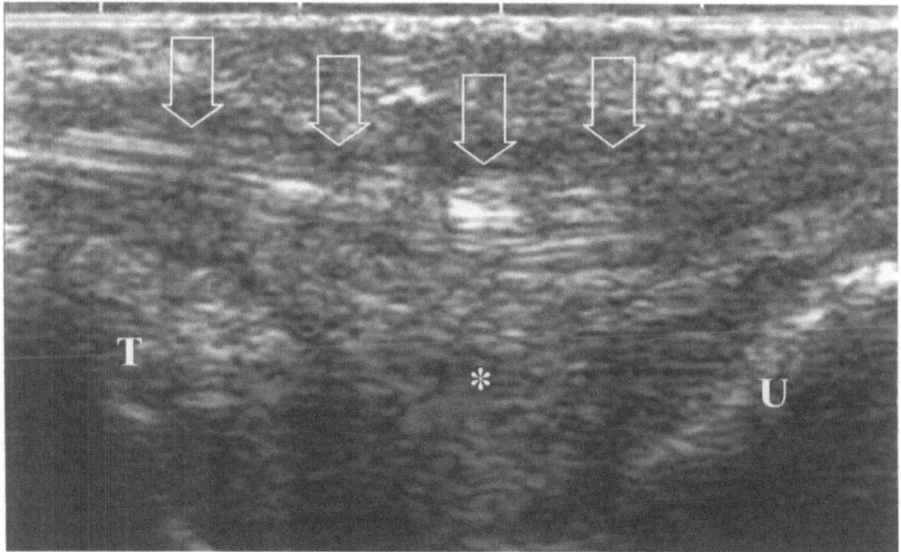

Fig. 24. Longitudinal scan of the dorsal aspect of the wrist near the styloid process. The TFC (asterisk) appears as a triangular hyperechoic structure located between the ulna (U) and the triquetrum (T), near the overlying extensor carpi ulnaris tendon (*arrows*)

anatomical landmark to visualize the TFC from the dorsal side of the wrist by longitudinal scans. Laterally to Lister's tuberculus, there are the extensor carpi radialis brevis and longus tendons and alongside the lateral surface of the distal epiphysis of the radius, the adductor longus and extensor pollicis brevis tendons (Fig. 26).

It is important to examine the surface of the carpal, metacarpal, and phalangeal bones, the articular hyaline cartilage, and the profile of the distal epiphysis of the radius and ulna, on top of which there are two synovial recesses. They are virtual in normal conditions and not visible at US; when enlarged by liquid and/or hypertrophic synovial membrane due to inflammation, they are easily distinguished by US.

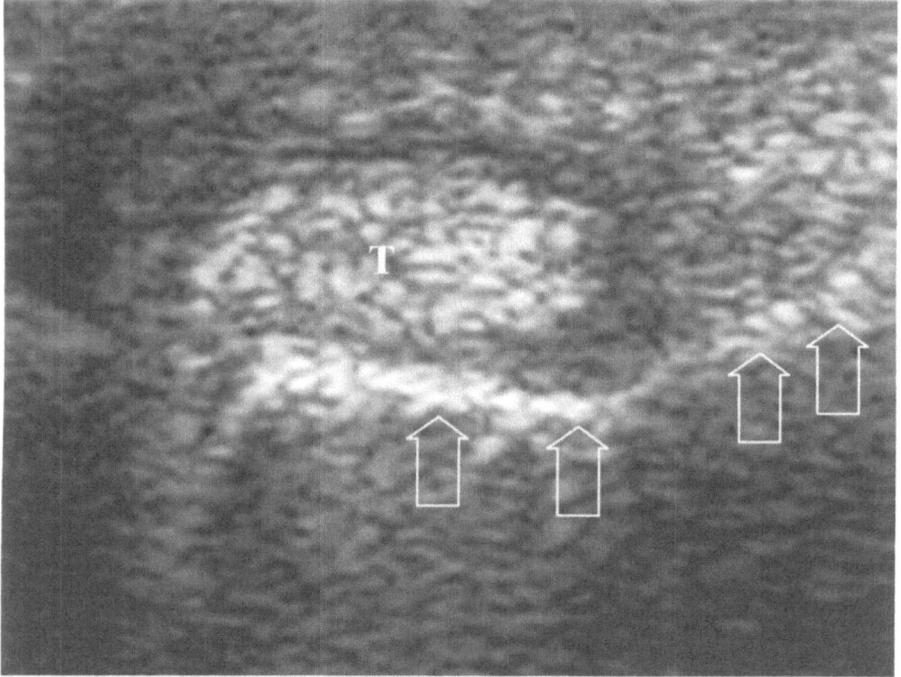

Fig. 25. Transverse scan of the dorsal aspect of the wrist near the styloid process. The extensor carpi ulnaris tendon is visible as a circular hyperechoic structure (*T*) located in a groove of the distal ulna (*arrows*)

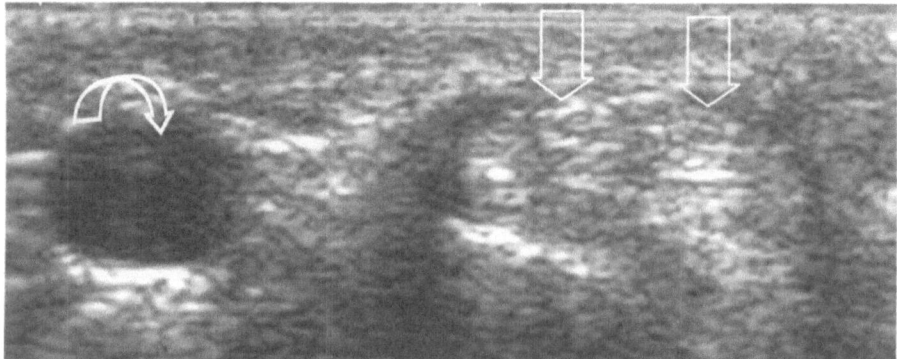

Fig. 26. Transverse scan of the lateral aspect of the wrist. The abductor longus and extensor pollicis brevis tendons are visible in this view (*arrows*). Laterally, the radial artery is also easily identified as an anechoic circular structure (*curved arrow*)

2.2.6 US in Rheumatoid Arthritis

US may recognize some of the early characteristics of the disease, such as intraarticular effusion, proliferation of synovial membrane, tenosynovitis, articular cartilage thinning, and marginal bone erosions.

Intraarticular effusion is a result of inflammation and not a specific finding. It is always associated with distension of the articular capsule and its synovial recesses. Effusion is usually anechoic, but may be hypoechoic due to fibrinosis (Fig. 27).

Synovial membrane involvement is more specific than simple effusion. At the beginning of the disease the deposition of fibrin on the synovial membrane gives an irregular appearance to the profile of the articular capsule and synovial recesses. When the disease is more advanced, there is an evident thickening of the synovial membrane due to its hypertrophy and hyperplasia, which may cause villosity protruding inside the articular cavity, with typical irregular US appearance (Fig. 28). In this phase it is not always easy to reach the diagnosis of synovial hyperplasia because of frequent contemporary joint effusion and significant fibrinosis. In this case transducer pressure on the examination area may be useful in order to move the fluid away and to identify the synovial proliferation. Alternatively the patient should move the wrist to allow differentiation of the liquid from the solid components.

Tenosynovitis is a frequent event in RA. The structures involved are the flexor and extensor tendons. The pathological appearance is characterized by direct involvement of the tendon, with widespread thickening, exudate, and proliferation of the tendon sheath. These alterations are reflected in typical US findings. The tendon is thickened and nonhomogeneous with loss of the normal fibrillar pattern (Fig. 29). If tenosynovitis is present, the tendon is surrounded by fluid, typically anechoic or hypoechoic and nonhomogeneous when containing fibrin or when associated

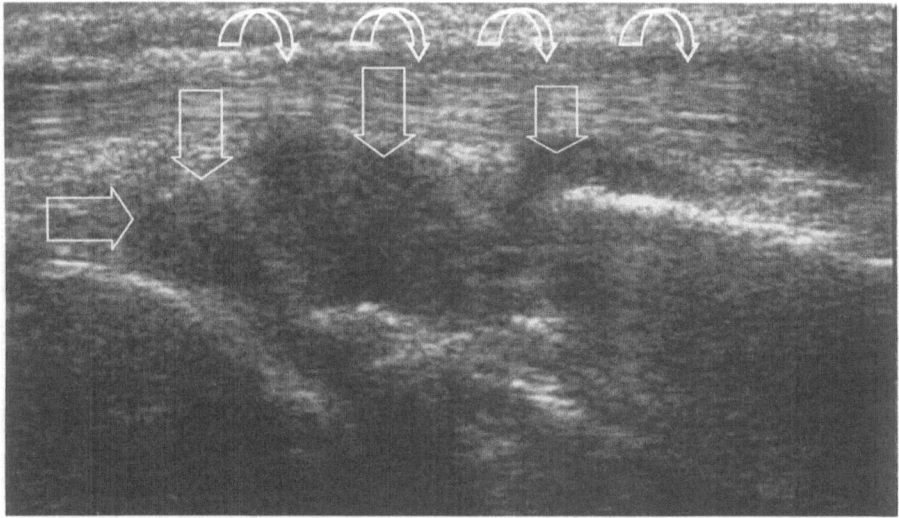

Fig. 27. Longitudinal scan of the dorsal aspect of the wrist at ulnar styloid process level. The synovial recess is distended by fluid with hypoechogenicity areas are due to the presence of fibrin (*arrows*). The extensor carpi ulnaris tendon sheath is also filled with fluid (*curved arrows*)

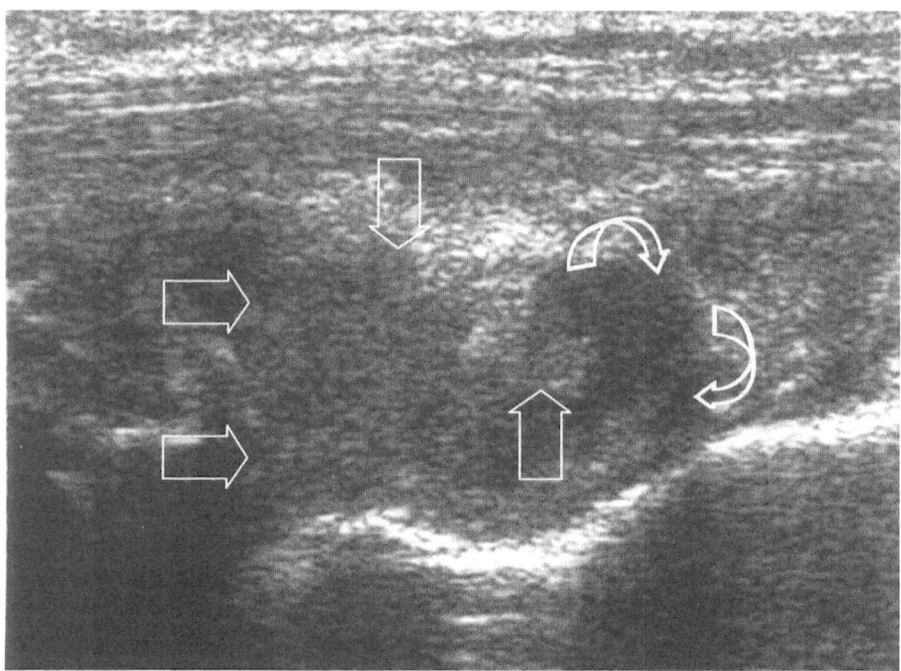

Fig. 28. Longitudinal scan of the volar aspect of the wrist at radiocarpal joint level. The anterior synovial recess is bulging. Synovial pannus is demonstrated in the joint space (*arrows*), surrounded by anechoic fluid (*curved arrows*)

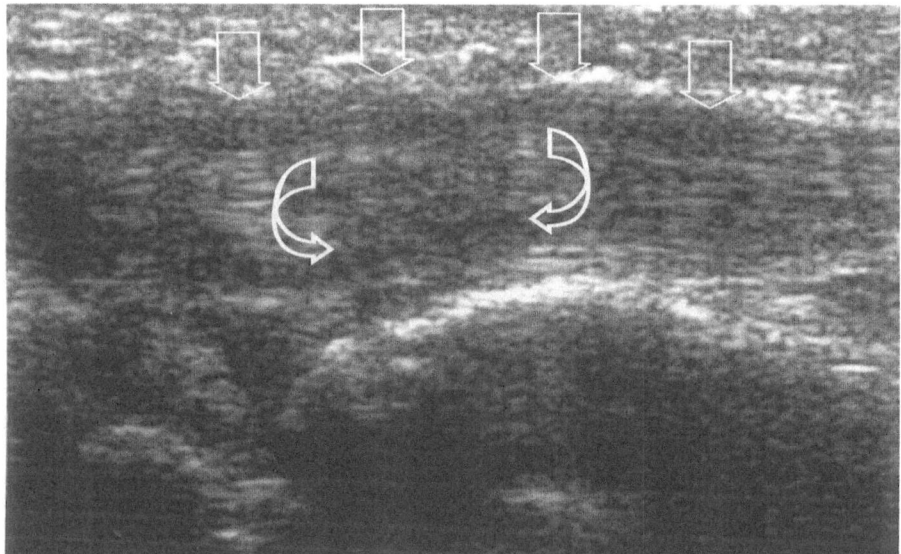

Fig. 29. Longitudinal scan of the anterior aspect of the wrist at carpal tunnel level. The flexor tendons sheath is slightly distended by inflammatory hypoechoic fluid (*arrows*). The tendons appear swollen and hypoechoic with disruption of their internal fibrillar network (*curved arrows*)

with synovial hyperplasia (Fig. 30). The final event of this process may be the pathological rupture of the tendon, easily recognizable as partial or complete interruption of the tendon structure (Fig. 31).

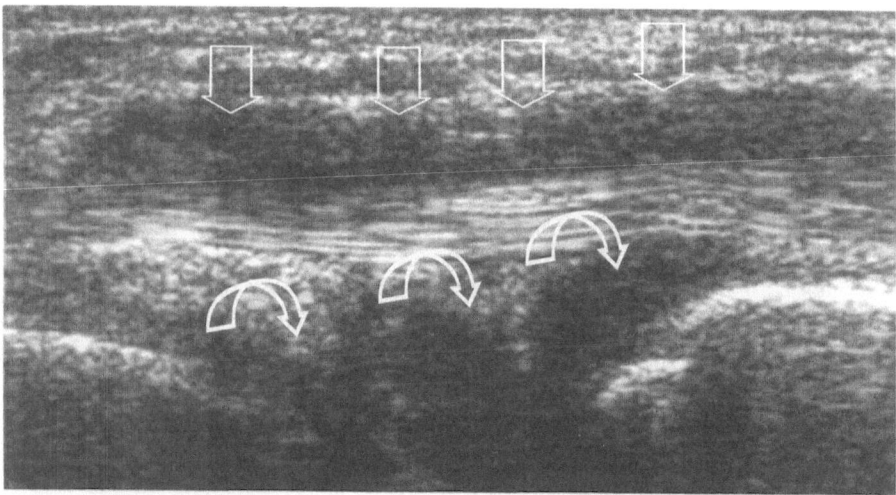

Fig. 30. Longitudinal scan of the dorsal aspect of the wrist at ulnar styloid process level. The extensor carpi ulnaris tendon sheath appears irregularly distended by inflammatory hypoechoic fluid (*arrows*) but no alterations of tendon echotexture are visible. The posterior synovial recess is also slightly filled by fluid (*curved arrows*)

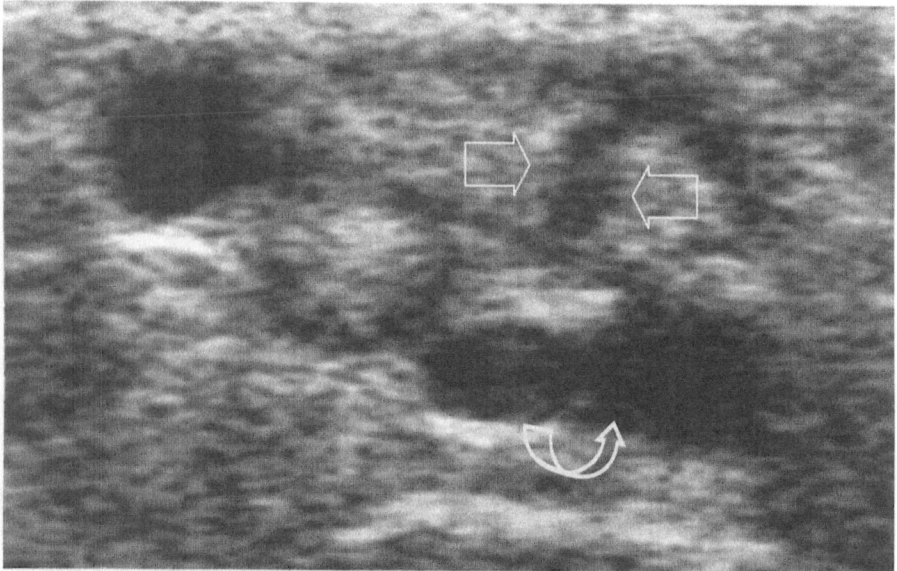

Fig. 31. Transverse scan of the dorsal aspect of the wrist at abductor pollicis longus and extensor pollicis brevis tendon level using a very high frequency transducer (20 MHz). The common sheath of the tendons appears distended by fluid (*curved arrow*). A small hypoechoic area of fibrillar fragmentation (*arrows*), suggestive of split lesion, is visible within the abductor pollicis longus tendon

US also allows appraisal of thinning of the articular cartilage and of marginal bone erosions, characterized, respectively, by a reduction of the usually regular and uniform thickness and by defects of the bone inside which it is possible to recognize the presence of synovial villosity, typically hypoechoic and nonhomogeneous (Fig. 32).

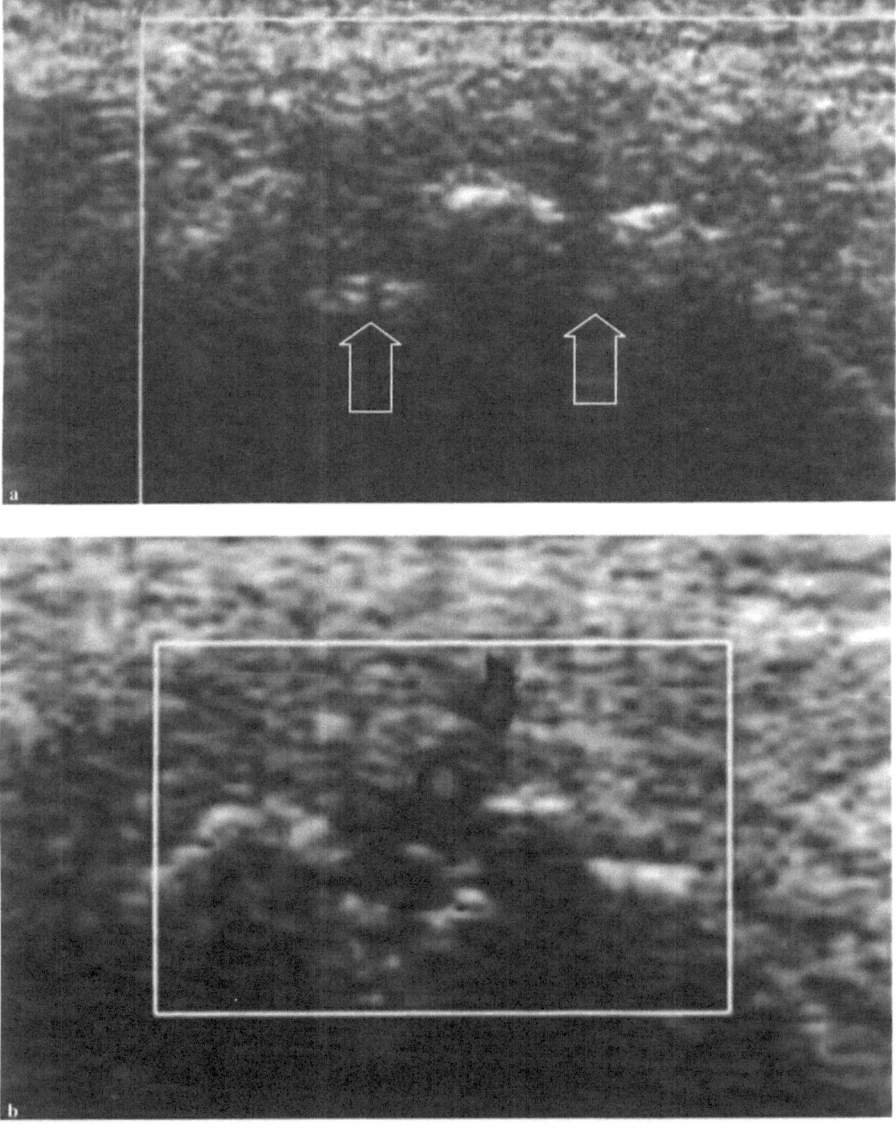

Fig. 32a, b. Transverse scans of the dorsal aspect of the wrist at capitatum bone level. **a** Some marginal erosions that interrupt the bone surface are visible (*arrows*). **b** PD US shows small flow signals within the synovial hypoechoic pannus that surrounds and fills these erosions

In contrast, US does not allow an adequate estimation of disease activity. In the active state, inflammatory hyperemia and neoangiogenetic processes are prevailing, followed by vascularized synovial proliferation. Thus it is necessary to complement standard US examination by color or power Doppler analysis. Power Doppler allows to distinguish also small vessels with slow flow and it is therefore the technique of choice for this kind of study. Recent studies have shown that power Doppler can recognize vascular signals in active synovial proliferation, as peripheral or centrally localized dot-like images, or as vascular structures longitudinally oriented (Figs. 33, 34). It is always important to complete the power Doppler evaluation with spectral analysis in order to avoid confusion between inflammatory vessels (typically low-resistance arterioles or venous vessels) and normal vessels of the cortical bone (high-resistance arterial vessels) (Figs. 35, 36). The evaluation of vessels in the hyperplastic synovial membrane allows, moreover, recognition of the synovial involvement of a joint effusion with a high rate of fibrin leakage by virtue of the internal flow signals (Fig. 37).

In the study of tenosynovitis it also seems useful to complete the examination with power Doppler. Flexor and extensor tendons all have tendon sheats with vessels localized in the mesotendium, parallel to the major tendon axis in order to allow the gliding of the visceral and parietal layers of the tendon sheath (Figs. 38, 39). Spectral analysis of vascular signals is essential in order to differentiate normal vessels (high resistance) from pathologically inflamed vessels (low resistance).

Power Doppler has proved to be a very useful technique in the follow-up of patients under medical therapy, because of its ability to clearly demonstrate a decrease in inflammation.

Nevertheless, besides the many advantages, there are well-defined limits to Doppler diagnostics, for instance, a nonquantitative evaluation of the state of inflammation and difficult technical reproducibility of the examination. Although technical limitations as well as difficulties in signal interpretation restrict the routine use of US contrast agents in the study of rheumatoid disease, it is important to remember that they allow a significant improvement in depicting slow flows (Fig. 40).

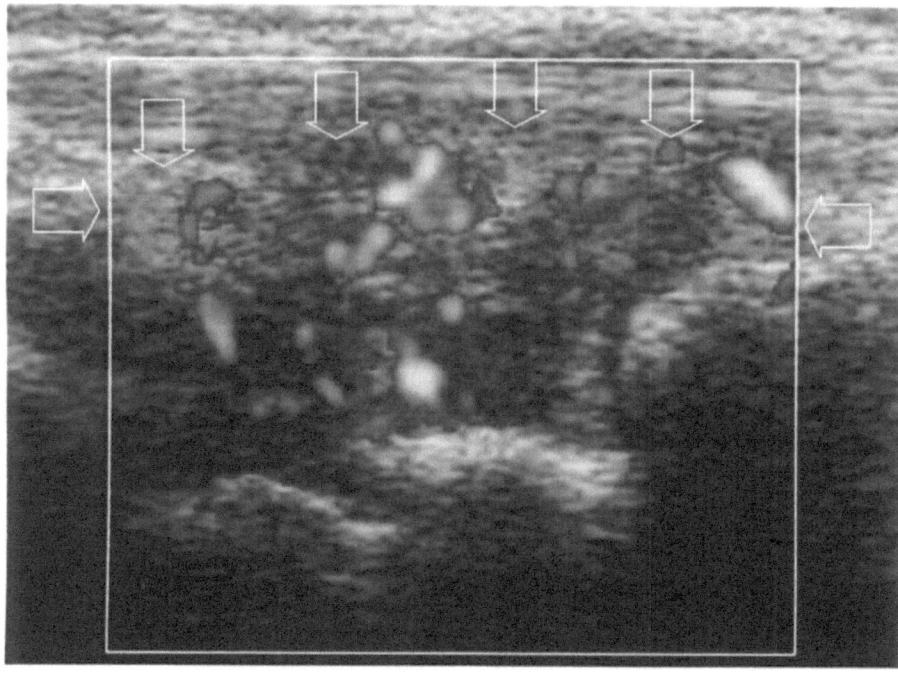

Fig. 33. Longitudinal scan of the dorsal aspect of the wrist near the ulnar styloid process. The posterior recess is bulging. PD US shows many flow spot signals that distribute at the periphery and inside the synovial pannus (*arrows*)

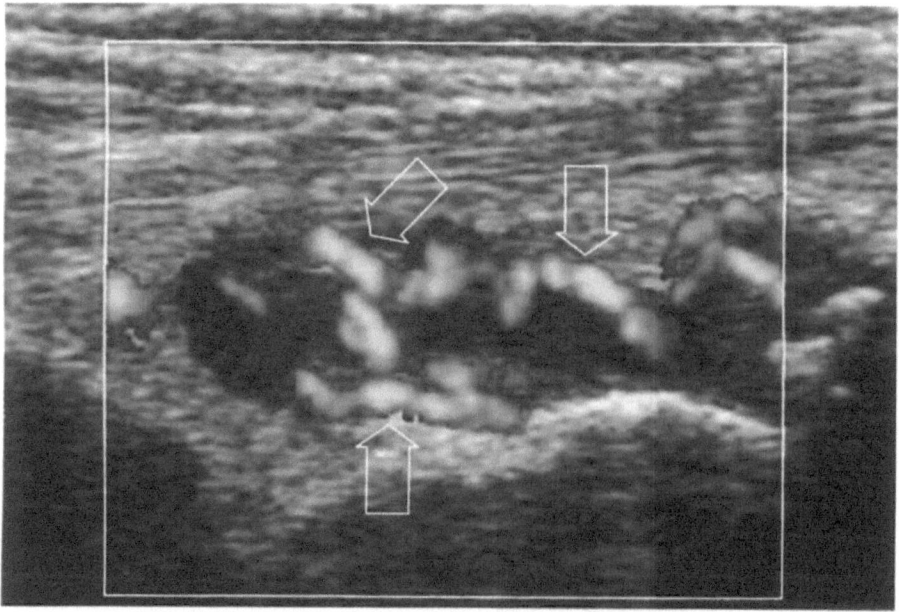

Fig. 34. Longitudinal scan of the wrist near the ulnar styloid process. PD US shows some vascular structures (*arrows*) that distribute longitudinally inside the synovial proliferation

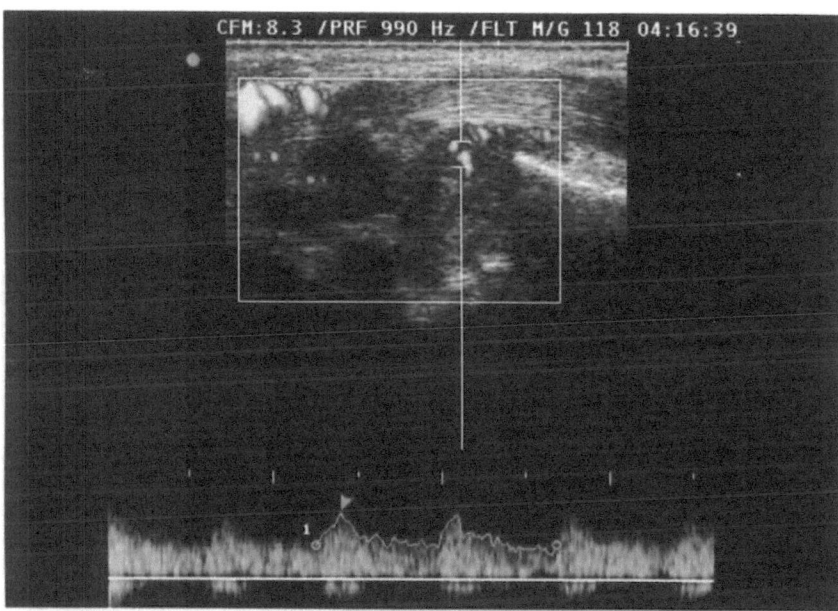

Fig. 35. Longitudinal scan of the volar aspect of the hand at the intercarpal joint level. Spectral analysis confirms the hyperemic origin of flow signals depicted by PD US. In this case it shows the waveform of a small artery with low resistance index (0.64)

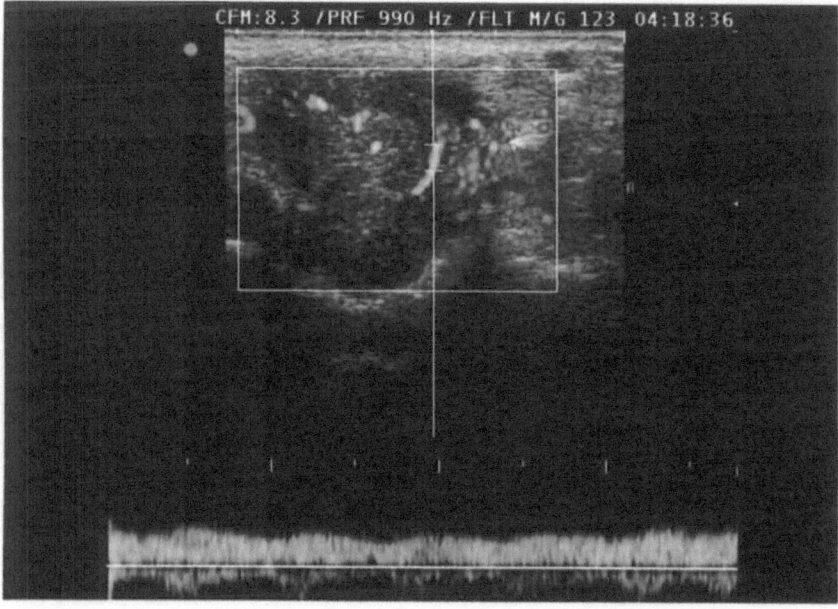

Fig. 36. Longitudinal scan of the volar aspect of the wrist near the flexor tendons of the second finger. PD US demonstrates some flow signals at tendon sheath level (that appears distended by inflammatory fluid and synovial pannus). Spectral analysis shows in this case the waveform of a small vein

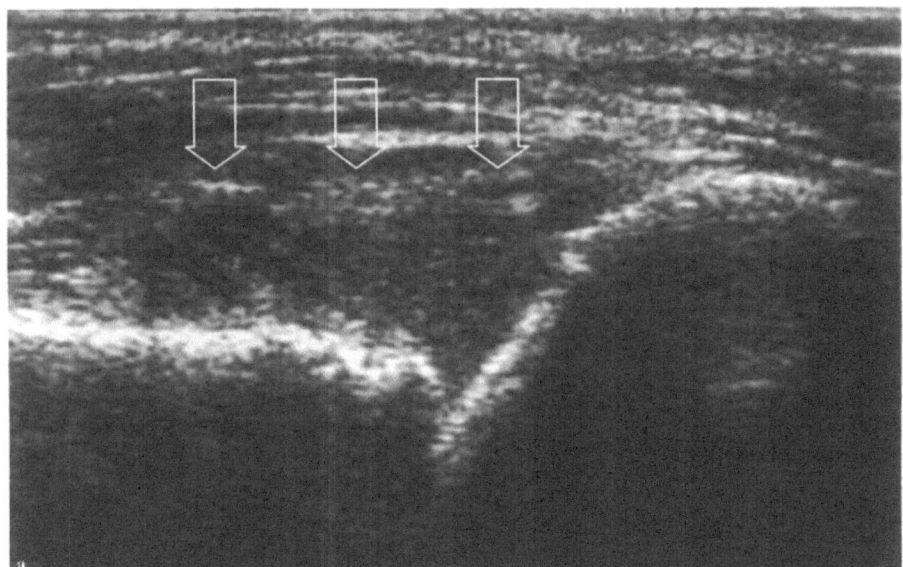

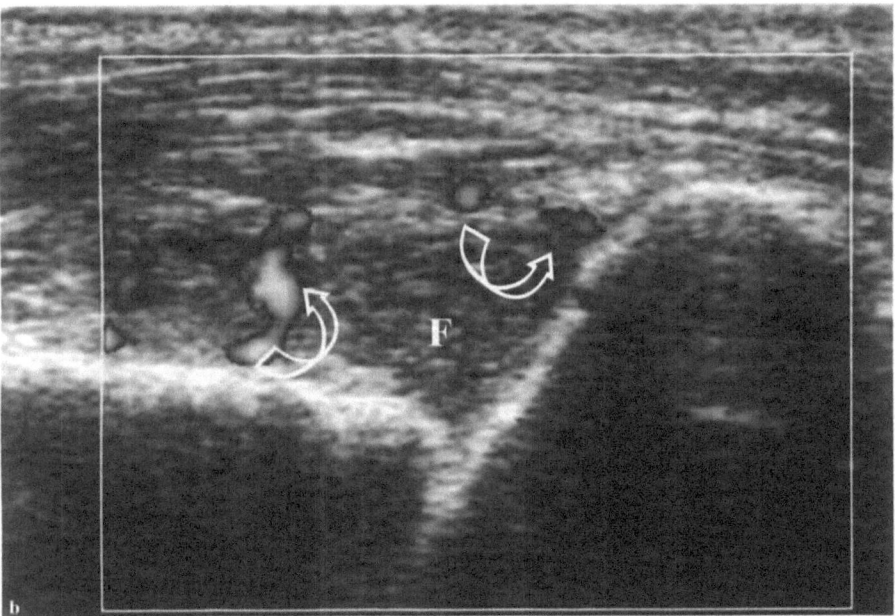

Fig. 37a, b. Longitudinal scans of the dorsal surface of the hand at the trapezoid-metacarpal joint level. **a** The joint capsule is distended by inflammatory fluid (*arrows*). It is not possible, on a B-mode image, to distinguish between fibrin and synovial proliferation. **b** PD US shows flow signals within the synovial pannus, thus helping to differentiate the peripheral proliferation (*curved arrows*) from fibrin (F)

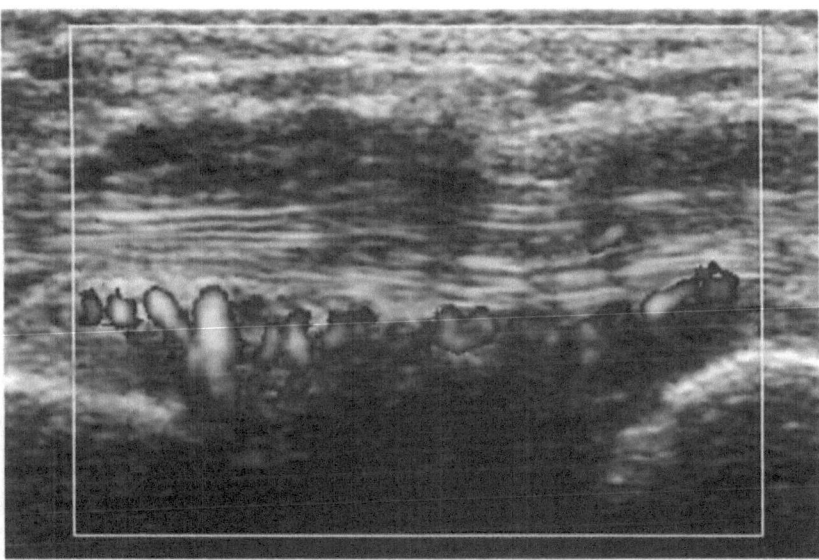

Fig. 38. Longitudinal scan of the dorsal surface of the wrist at the ulnar styloid process level. PD US shows some flow spot signals within the extensor ulnaris carpi tendon sheath

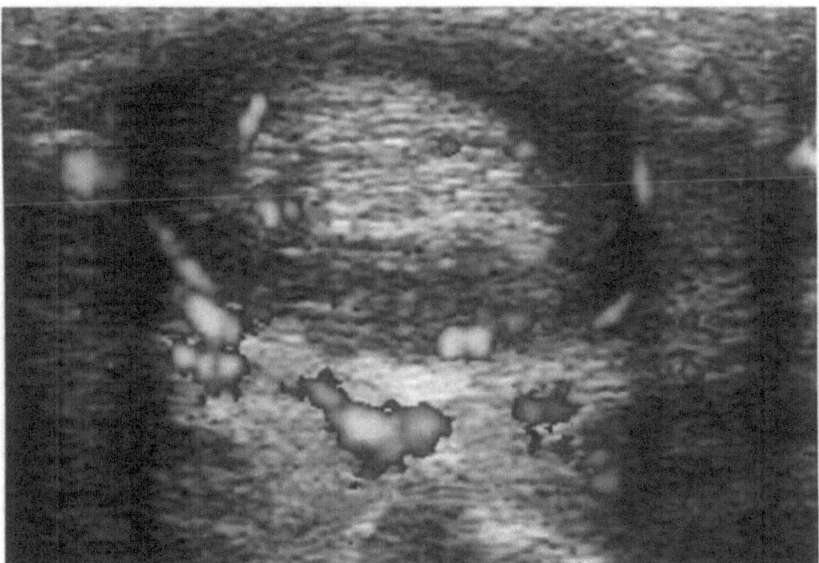

Fig. 39. Transverse scan of the volar aspect of the hand in a patient affected by rheumatoid tenosynovitis of flexor tendons of the third finger. In this case PD US depicts vascular structures at the tendon sheath level

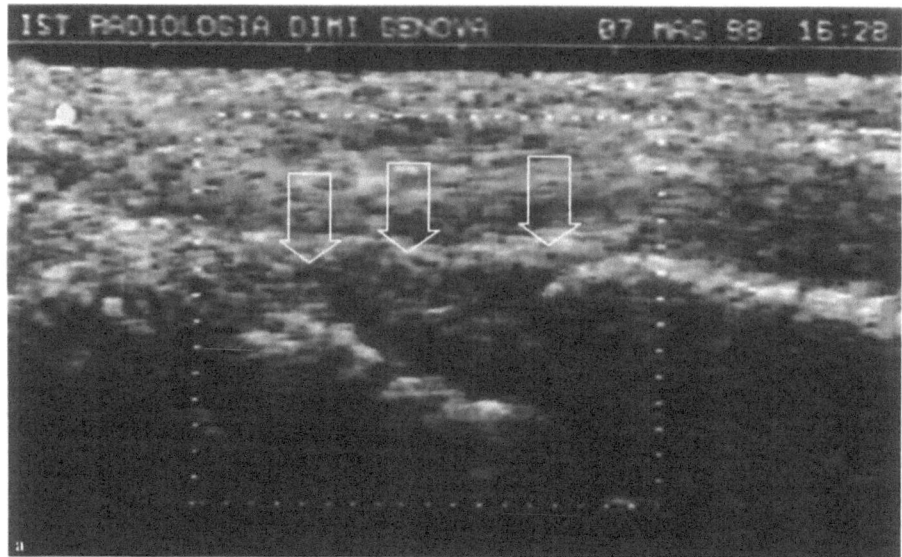

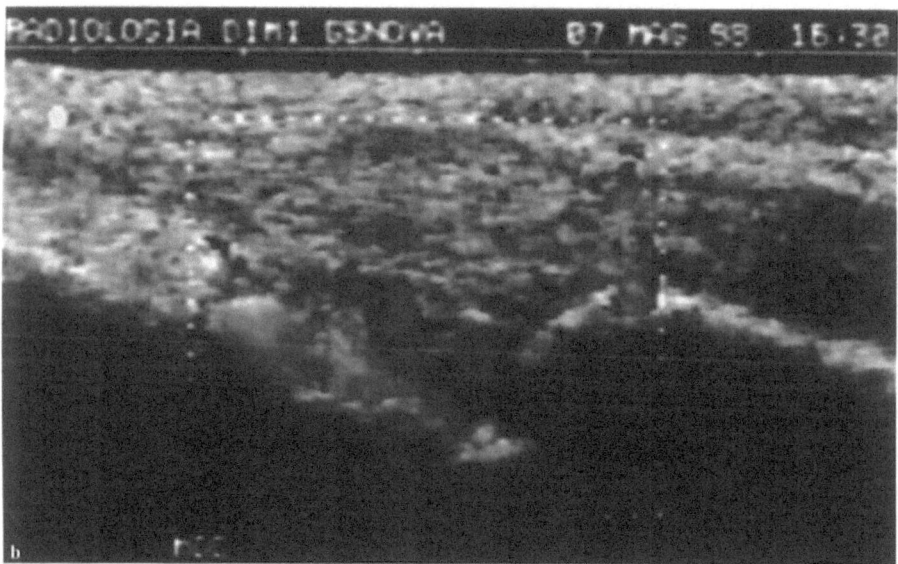

Fig. 40a, b. Longitudinal scans of the dorsal surface of the wrist near the ulnar styloid process obtained before (**a**) and after (**b**) the intravenous administration of an US contrast agent. **a** In basal condition, PD US does not show any flow signals within the synovial proliferation (*arrows*). **b** After the injection of the contrast agent some flow signals are visible, especially on the carpal side (images taken from a videotape)

2.3   Magnetic Resonance

The hand is one of the most difficult anatomical areas to investigate because of the small dimensions of the different structures (bones, ligaments, tendons, and nerves) organized in a limited space.

Thanks to its high resolution and contrast capabilities, an exhaustive analysis of all the structures of the hand, can be performed with MR.

Therefore MR is increasingly used for studying those pathologies such as RA whose early alterations are typical of this region. Moreover, there is the possibility of monitoring disease activity with the use of paramagnetic contrast agents.

The availability of low-field (0.2 T) MR units dedicated to the examination of limb joints yields significant advantages in comparison with whole body MR systems. The cost/benefit ratio is so favorable (see Table 7) to induce us (except in some selected or difficult to interpret cases) to use dedicated MR systems in the evaluation of rheumatoid patients.

Regardless of the choice between "whole body" and "dedicated" systems, more relevant is the optimization of study techniques. This includes acquisition matrix, slice thickness, field of view, signal-to-noise ratio, choice of sequences, number of acquisitions, etc. An optimal compromise among all these parameters and acquisition time is necessary to obtain good and highly diagnostic images, and for the correct evaluation of rheumatic disease since their earliest manifestations.

Table 7. Advantages of dedicated MR systems

- Low purchase, setup and maintenance costs

- Small size

- Medium- to low-intensity magnetic field

- Developed specifically for small joints (e.g., wrist and hand) with adequate field of view (FOV) and homogeneity calculated for the anatomical region of interest

- Spatial resolution and optimized sequences to interpret most of the clinical questions in rheumatoid arthritis

- Excellent patient compliance and absence of claustrophobia

- Ability to examine patients with prostheses or metallic implants (not in the examination field)

2.3.1   Examination Technique

Using a dedicated MR unit, the examination can be divided into three standardized phases: positioning of the limb, setup of examination data, and acquisition of sequences.

The examination starts with positioning of the limb in the dedicated coil (Fig. 41).

The area to be investigated has to be strictly positioned in the receiving coil center in the middle of the magnet. This is an easy but critical operation due to the ex-

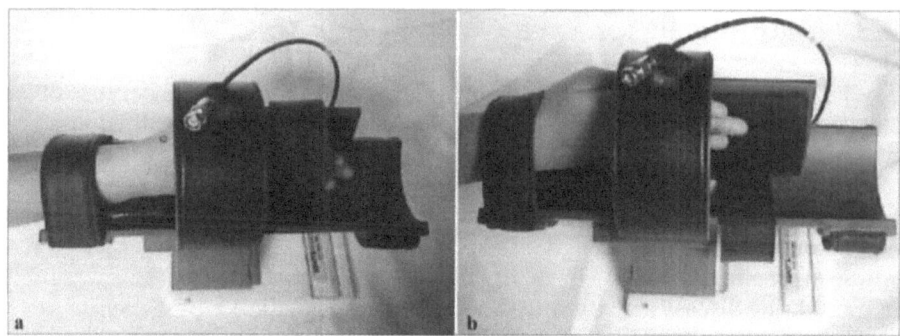

Fig. 41a, b. Positioning of the patient's limb in the dedicated coil. In the wrist examination (**a**) the lower limit of the anatomical snuff-box has to be positioned in correspondence to the internal border of the coil. In the hand examination (**b**) the extremity of the distal phalanx of the third finger has to be positioned in correspondence to the external border of the coil

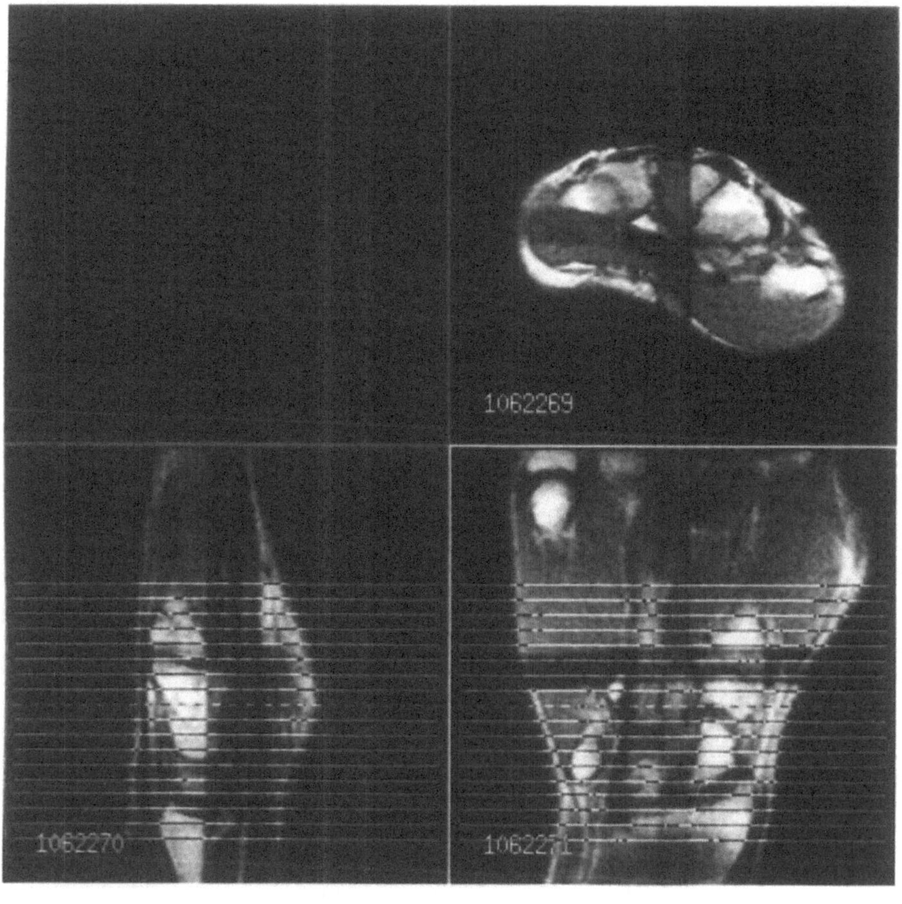

Fig. 42. "Scout" images. These images in axial, sagittal, and coronal planes are important for verifying the correct joint positioning inside the magnet and as a reference for the following acquisitions

tension of the magnetic field of view (FOV) of 12 cm, smaller than in whole body units but wide enough to examine the region of interest.

The positioning phase is immediately followed by examination data setup and acquisition of three "scout" images in axial, sagittal, and coronal planes. These images are extremely important to verify the correct joint positioning inside the magnet and are used for the acquisition planning (Fig. 42). Finally, specific sequence protocols are chosen according to the pathology.

2.3.2 MR Normal Anatomy

2.3.2.1 Bone

Independent of the sequence, a total lack of signal from both cortical and trabecular bone is observed (Fig. 43).

2.3.2.2 Bone Marrow

Bone marrow shows a signal highly dependent on the type of marrow: red or yellow. In red marrow, a higher concentration of blood lengthens the relaxation times, resulting in a slightly hypointense signal in T1-weighted sequences and a hyperintense signal in T2-weighted sequences. Shorter relaxation times in yellow marrow, in which the adipose component is higher, cause the signal to be mildly higher in T1-weighted sequences and relatively reduced in T2-weighted sequences (Fig. 44).

2.3.2.3 Hyaline Cartilage

In hyaline cartilage water is bound to the collagen fibers, and its concentration and mobility change in the different layers.

Generally cartilage shows moderate hyperintensity in T1-weighted sequences, while its signal is reduced in T2-weighted sequences (Fig. 45).

2.3.2.4 Tendons, Ligaments and Joint Capsule

These structures, rich in collagen, have so fast relaxation times that they do not allow adequate signal discrimination in all T1- and T2-weighted sequences, hence resulting in marked signal hypointensity (Fig. 46). When collagen fibers are oriented in the magnetic field at about 55°, the "magic angle effect" takes place, resulting in an elongation of T2 relaxation time of collagen, with a consequent signal increase in T1-weighted images.

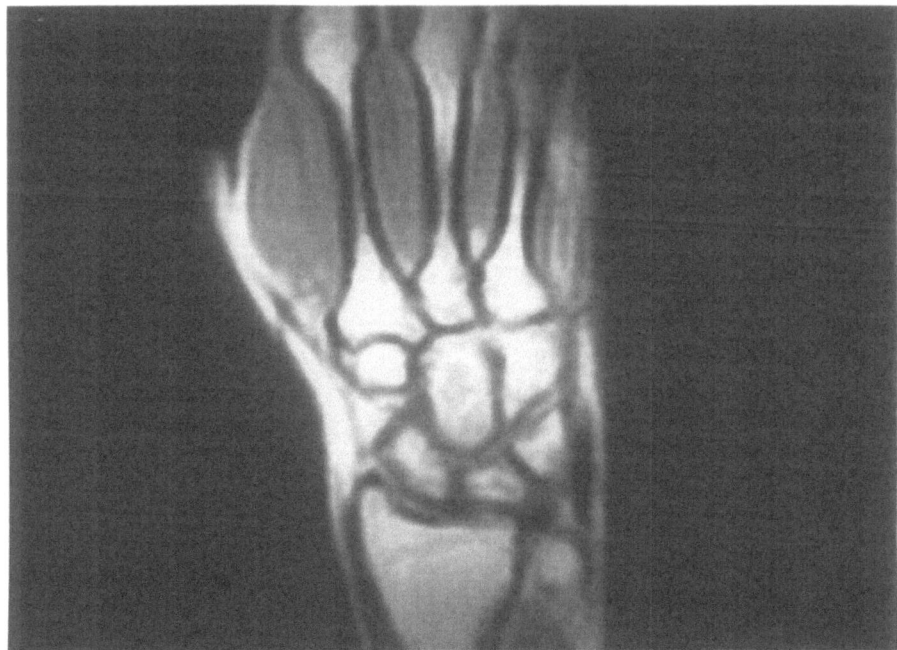

Fig. 43. T1-weighted coronal spin echo (SE) image of the wrist. A total lack of signal from cortical bone, which is markedly hypointense, is seen

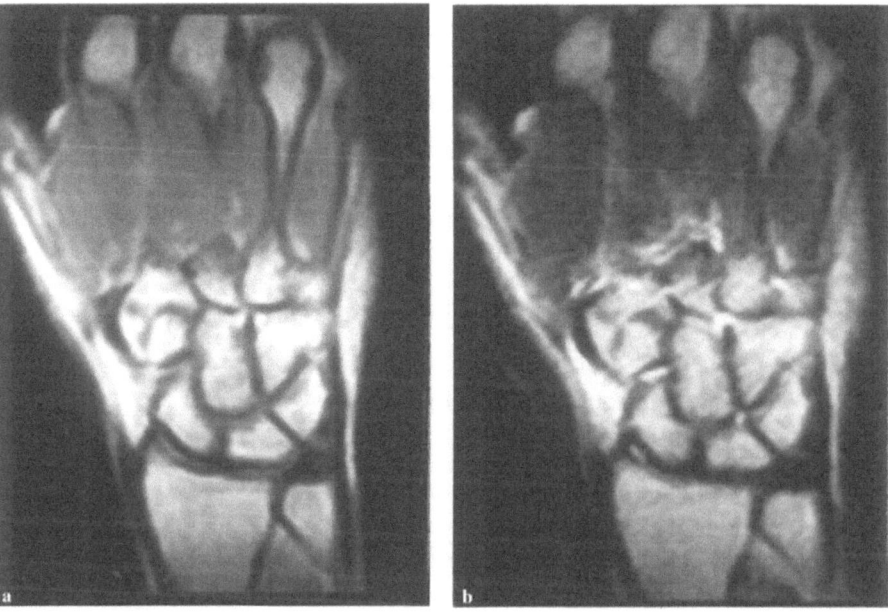

Fig. 44a, b. T1-weighted (**a**) and T2-weighted (**b**) coronal SE images. Good depiction of yellow marrow, which is characterized by moderate signal hyperintensity in T1-weighted sequences and relatively reduced signal intensity in T2-weighted ones

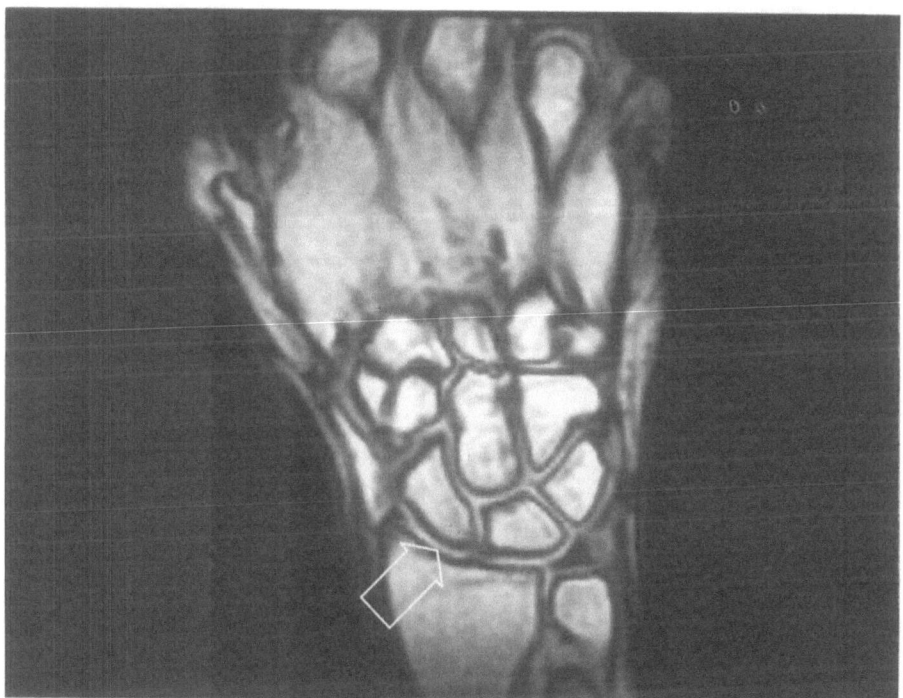

Fig. 45. T1-weighted coronal gradient echo (GE) image. Hyaline cartilage appears moderately hyperintense (*arrow*)

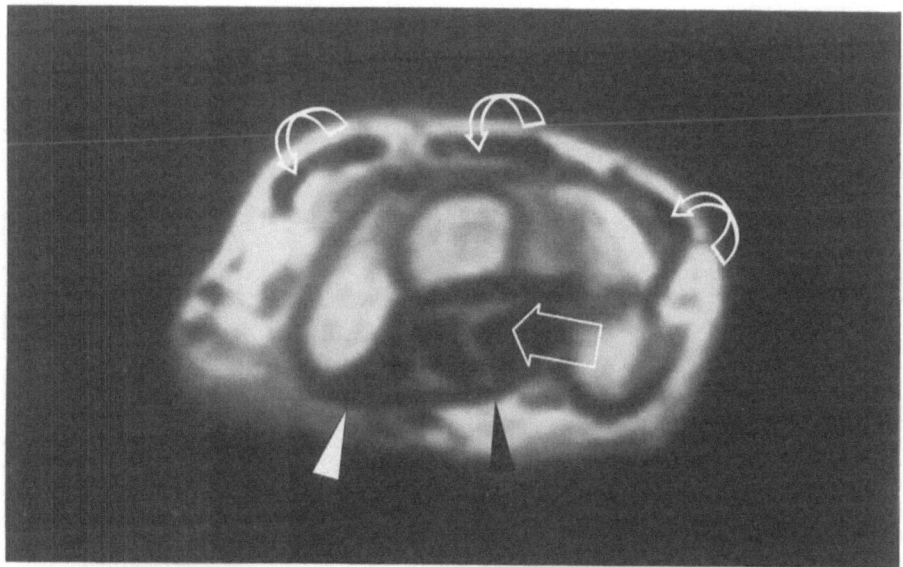

Fig. 46. A T1-weighted axial SE image shows the normal low signal intensity of flexor tendons (*straight arrow*), flexor retinaculum (*arrowheads*) and extensor tendons (*curved arrows*)

2.3.2.5 Muscular Tissue

In muscular tissue, water molecules are bound to cellular macromolecules inside the fibers, presenting moderately short relaxation times, which in T1-weighted sequences means modest signal hypointensity and in T2-weighted sequences, marked hypointensity (Fig. 47).

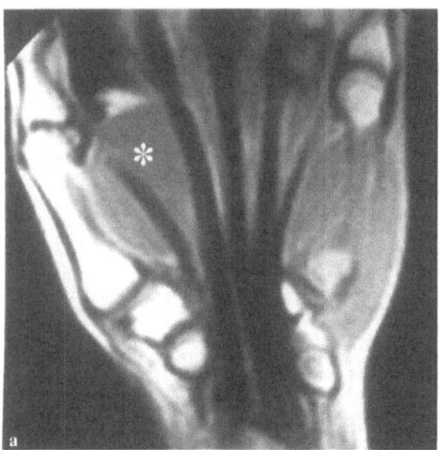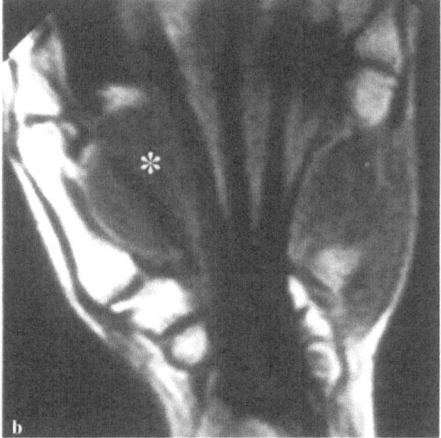

Fig. 47a, b. T1-weighted (**a**) and T2-weighted (**b**) coronal SE images. Muscular tissue appears modestly hypointense in the T1-weighted sequence (*asterisk*) and markedly hypointense in the T2-weighted one (*asterisk*)

2.3.2.6 Adipose Tissue

Adipose tissue is characterized by fast relaxation times, showing marked signal hyperintensity in T1-weighted sequences and relatively reduced signal intensity in T2-weighted sequences (Fig. 48).

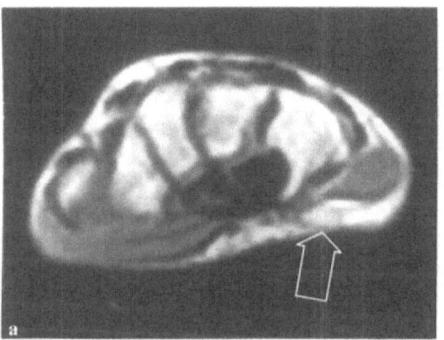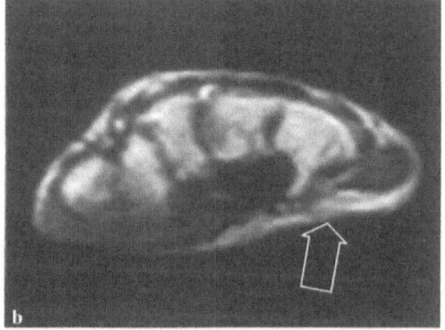

Fig. 48a, b. T1-weighted (**a**) and T2-weighted (**b**) axial SE images. Adipose tissue is characterized by signal hyperintensity in the T1-weighted sequence and relatively reduced signal intensity in the T2-weighted one (*arrow*)

2.3.2.7 Fluids

Fluids contain mainly water molecules, extremely mobile when free from molecular binding; this results in long relaxation times and hypointense signal in T1-weighted sequences and markedly hyperintense signal in T2-weighted sequences.

In the case of synovial inflammatory fluid, because of the higher content of water bound to proteic macromolecules, the protonic relaxation time is significantly shorter with consequent marked signal hyperintensity both T1- and T2-weighted sequences (Fig. 49).

A protocol commonly used in the examination of the rheumatoid hand is shown. According to our experience of about 1500 RA examinations, this protocol provides an accurate evaluation of alterations in synovial membrane, tendons, ligaments, cartilage, and bone (Table 8).

As stated above, the best compromise between signal to noise, spatial resolution, and contrast resolution is the objective of this protocol. The key point is the acquisition time, which must be kept as short as possible, especially when dealing with pa-

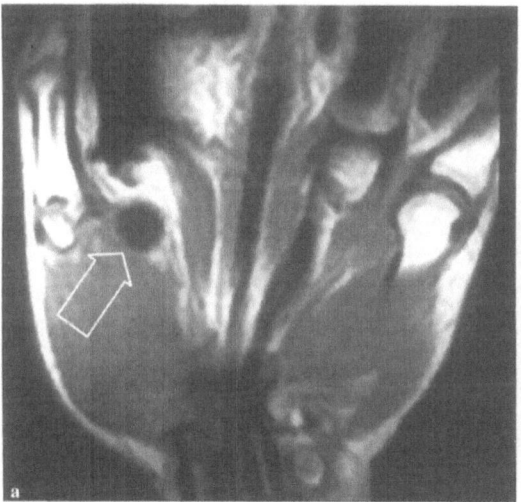 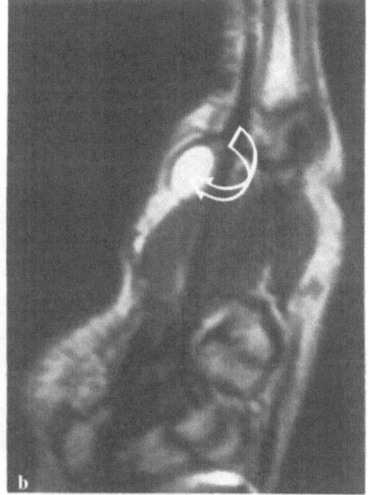

Fig. 49a, b. A T1-weighted (**a**) coronal SE image shows a synovial cyst (*straight arrow*), hypointense in signal and sharply marginated, adjacent to the first finger flexor tendon. A T2-weighted (**b**) SE sagittal image demonstrates the fluid content of the lesion, characterized by marked signal hyperintensity (*curved arrow*)

Table 8. MR protocol for rheumatoid wrist and hand examination

Sequence	TR/TE	Thickness	FOV	Matrix	NEX
GE T1-w	520/16	3.5	160×160	192×160	3
STIR	1300/24/85	3.5	200×170	192×160	2
SE T1-w	540/20	3.5	160×160	192×160	3
3D	30/12	1.4	200×170×100	192×160×72	1

Scans in coronal and axial relative planes for the carpus and coronal for the hand

tients with painful syndromes, in order to avoid motion artifacts. In these cases a single acquisition sequence may be performed, increasing the FOV to 170 mm in order to slightly increase the signal-to-noise ratio. As already discussed, the clinical value of the acquired images is the result of this compromise, and not related simply to one of the involved parameters.

2.3.3   Magnetic Resonance in Rheumatoid Arthritis

In the evaluation of RA, MR gives diagnostic information essential for a more accurate quantification of articular damage. From a radiological point of view, three well-differentiated phases in RA are distinguishable: synovial, synovial-cartilaginous and ankylosing.

In the **synovial phase**, the synovial membrane becomes, hyperplastic, and infiltrated by inflammatory cells (synovial pannus) with an increase of the synovial fluid. The synovial pannus is locally invasive, causing progressive erosion of articular cartilage and subchondral bone. The synovial membrane, normally regular and thin, in this phase becomes thickened with a villous appearance involving the areas not covered by articular cartilage. Therefore, synovial membrane hypertrophy, effusion, and pannus are the most important findings of the onset of RA.

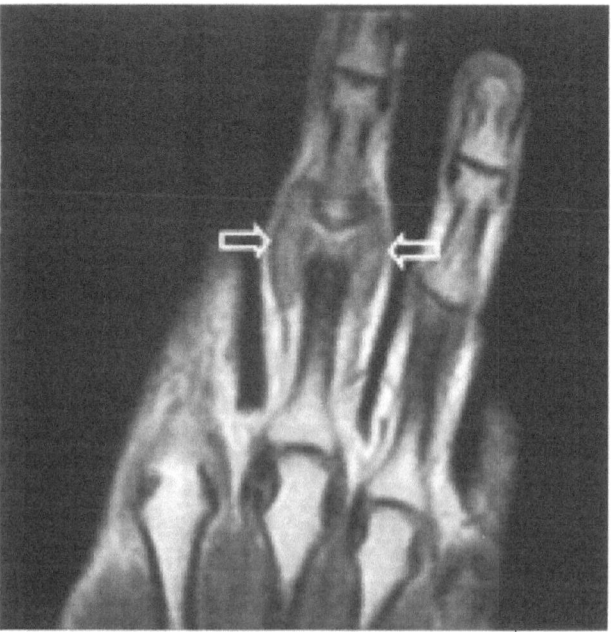

Fig. 50. MR scan of the right hand, T1-weighted coronal SE image. Synovial membrane swelling with overdistension of third finger proximal interphalangeal joint capsule due to the presence of heterogeneously hypointense tissue (*arrows*)

MR gives the possibility of clearly identifying the pathological changes of the synovial phase. These range from synovial membrane hypertrophy, with thickening of joint capsule (Fig. 50), to the presence of intraarticular effusion *(hyperintense in SE T2-weighted and STIR sequences* – Fig. 51), and synovial pannus formation *(slightly hypointense in SE T1-weighted and STIR sequences* – Fig. 52).

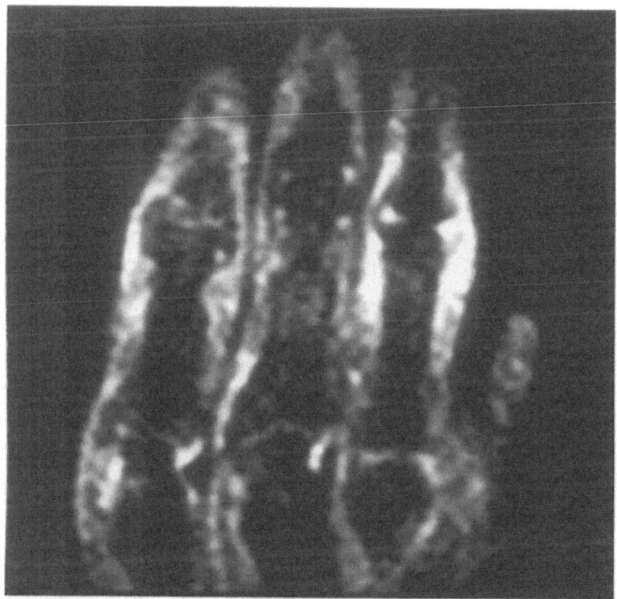

Fig. 51. MR scan of the right hand, coronal short tau inversion recovery (STIR) image. Intraarticular effusion, markedly hyperintense, at the level of the PIP joint in the fourth finger

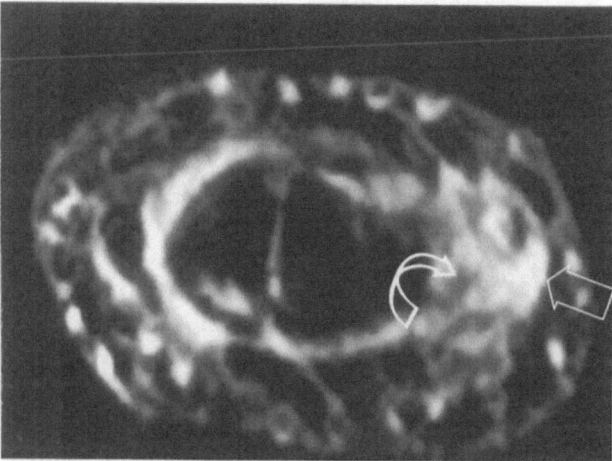

Fig. 52. Axial STIR image. Synovial involvement of the ulnar aspect of the wrist. The STIR sequence allows identification of both liquid effusion (hyperintense – *straight arrow*) and synovial pannus formation (hypointense – *curved arrow*)

The synovial phase is followed by the **synovial-cartilaginous phase**, characterized by inflammatory tissue invasion of articular cartilage, with slow and progressive destruction; infiltration of subchondral bone with cysts and bone erosions is easily demonstrated by MR with *GE T1-weighted* sequences, followed by *STIR* sequences (Figs. 53, 54).

A further evolution of the disease leads to the progressive disappearance of the joint space and the production of fibrous tissue, sometimes partially ossified, that joins the opposing epiphyses. Subluxation or permanent luxation (**ankylosing phase**) can also occur. MR readily demonstrates the morphostructural alterations typical of this phase (Fig. 55).

RA involvement of extraarticular synovial membranes that line bursae and tendon sheaths is well demonstrated by MR (Figs. 56, 57).

Far more complicated, is the analysis of the state of "activity" or "rest" of the rheumatoid process. MR with paramagnetic contrast agents enables the distinction of the active synovial pannus from the areas of resting or fibrotic synovia. The MR parameters, the methods for contrast agent administration, the sequences and the acquisition times we use for the evaluation of the state of activity of the disease are shown in Table 9 and Fig. 58.

Until recently, follow-up of patients affected by RA was based only on clinical and laboratory findings, and conventional radiography. In our Center for Imaging of Arthropathies and in other centers throughout the world, studies to validate the use of MR in the follow-up of patients with RA are in progress. In particular, a recent method for synovitis evaluation studies the degree of synovial pannus en-

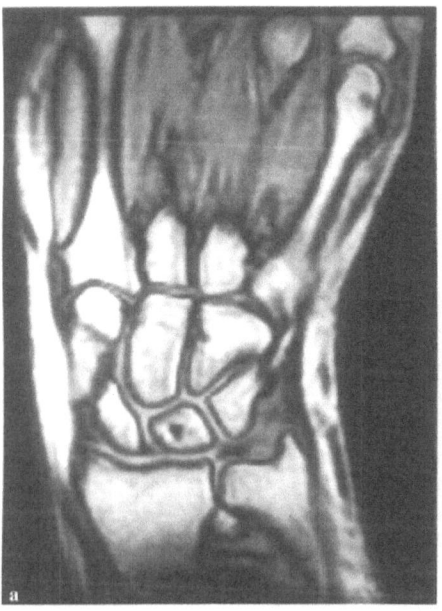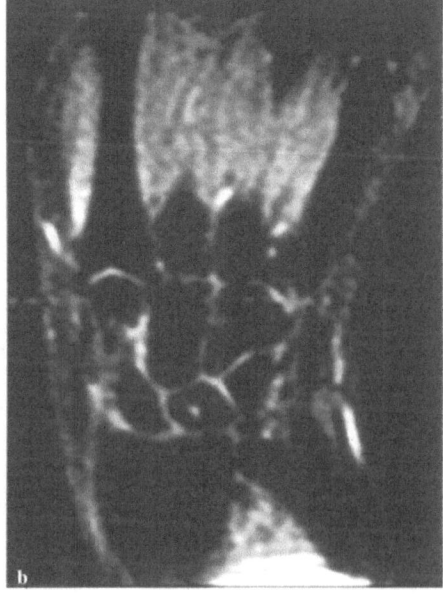

Fig. 53a, b. T1- weighted coronal GE (**a**) and STIR images (**b**). An intraosseous cyst at the center of the lunate demonstrates hypointensity in the T1-weighted sequence and hyperintensity in the STIR sequence

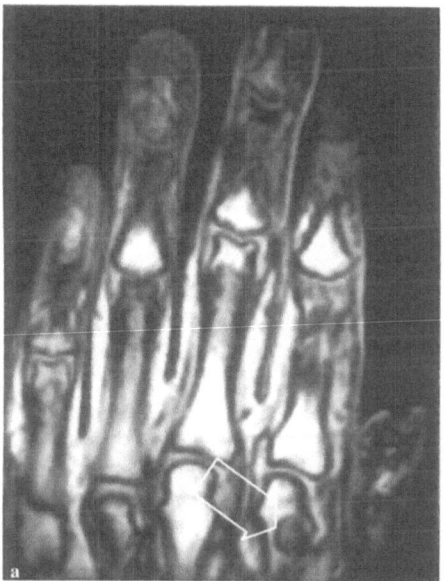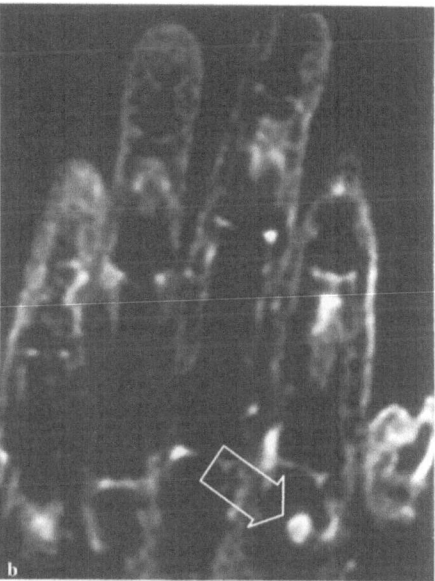

Fig. 54a, b. T1-weighted coronal GE image (**a**). A bone erosion (*arrow*) is appreciable at the level of the second metacarpal head of the left hand. On a STIR sequence (**b**) the lesion appears markedly hyperintense due to the presence of synovial membrane and/or fluid

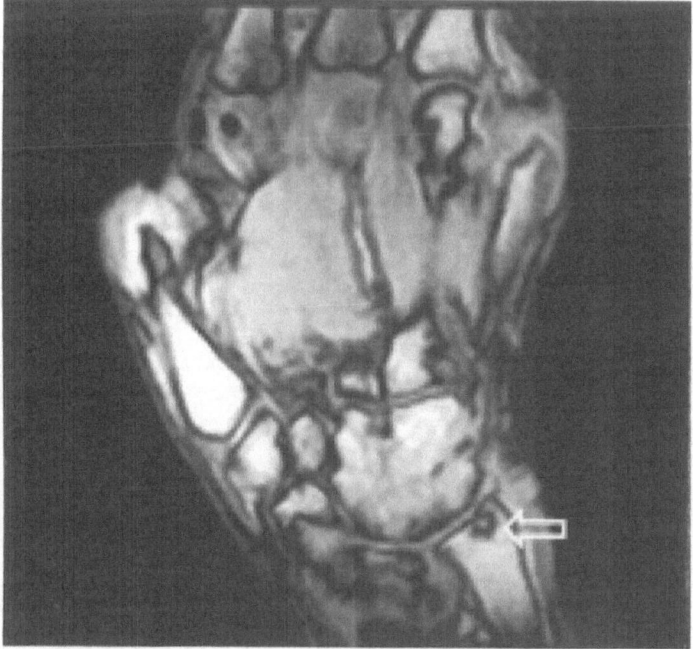

Fig. 55. A T1-weighted coronal GE sequence shows bone fusion involving the lunate, triquetrum and hamate. An erosion of the ulnar styloid is also present (*arrow*)

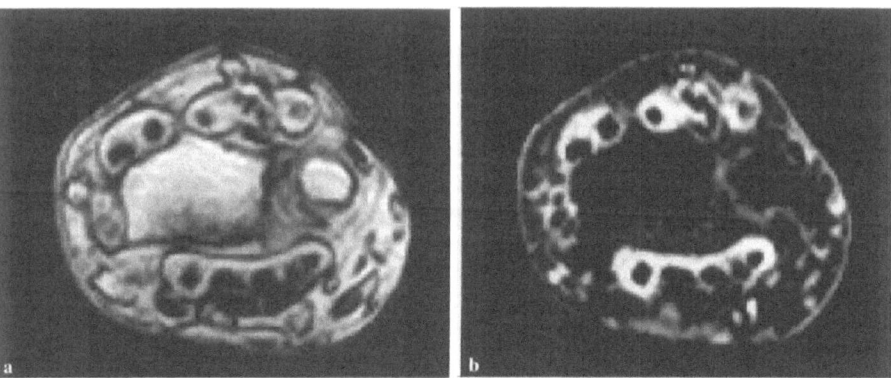

Fig. 56a, b. MR scans with axial GE T1-weighted (**a**) and STIR (**b**) sequences. MR shows tenosynovitis of the extensor tendons (in particular extensor carpi radialis brevis and longus, extensor pollicis longus and extensor digiti minimi) and of the flexor tendons (flexor pollicis and deep flexors of fingers)

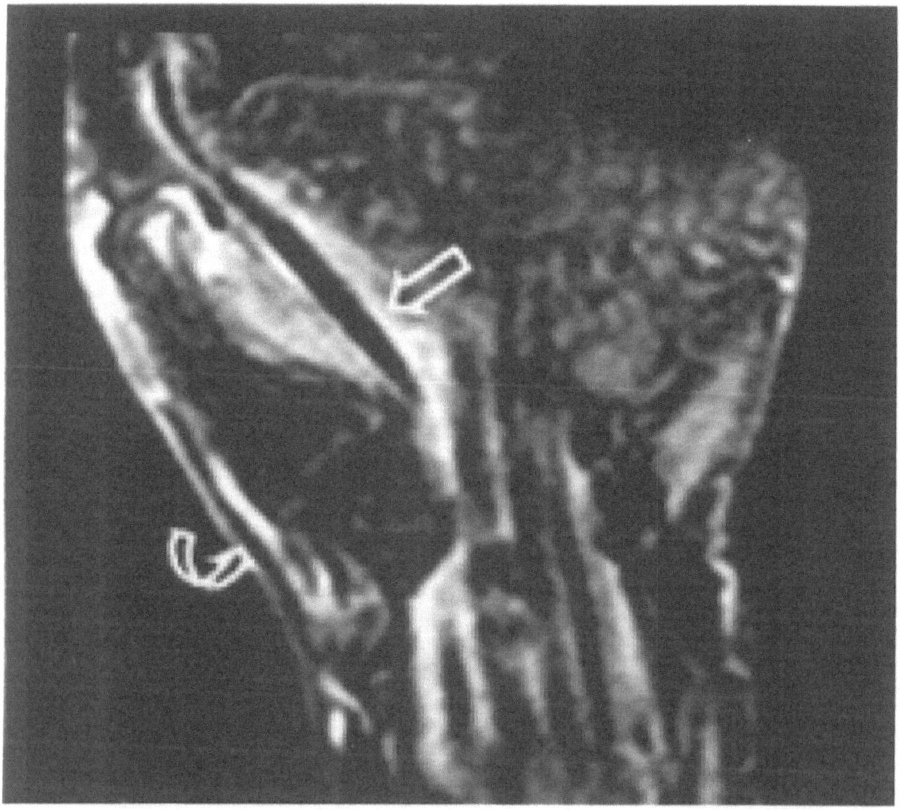

Fig. 57. MR scan with coronal STIR sequence. MR shows tenosynovitis of flexor pollicis longus (*straight arrow*) and of the corresponding extensor tendon (*curved arrow*). The tendons, which contain no water, do not provide any signal and therefore appear black. They are surrounded by the tendon sheath that appears white due to the presence of inflammation and effusion

Table 9. MR examination protocol for the rheumatoid wrist and hand using paramagnetic contrast agent (c.a.)

Sequence	TR/TE	Thickness	FOV	Matrix	NEX
SE T1-w	110/24	5/0.5	180×180	192×160	3

Pre-contrast sequence for the radiocarpal joint on axial planes

Paramagnetic c.a. administered intravenously in bolus (0.2 mmol/kg of body weight)

Intervals of repetition of the same sequence post-contrast: End of injection – 1 min – 2 min – 3 min – 4 min – 5 min – 10 min

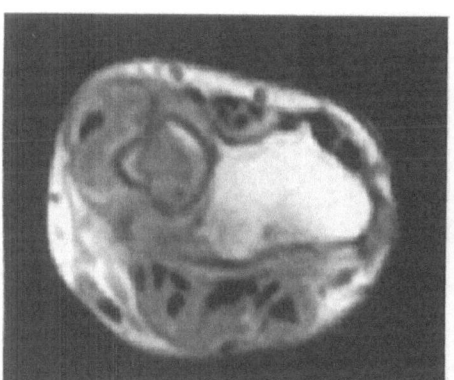 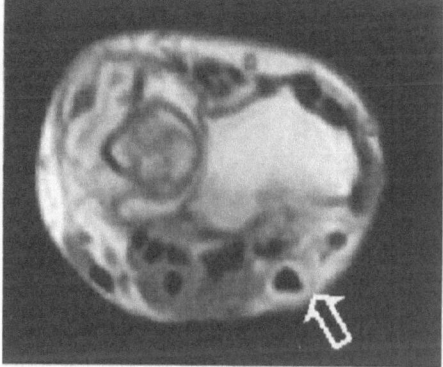

Fig. 58a, b. Axial MR scans with SE T1-weighted (pre- and post-contrast) sequences. Pre-contrast scans (**a**) show synovial involvement, more evident on the ulnar aspect, but provide a poor differentiation between fluid effusion and synovial membrane proliferation; "direct" MR does not allow an analysis of the degree of activity of RA. After contrast injection (**b**) a marked increase of signal intensity becomes evident, an expression of phenomenon of phlogistic hyperemia and neoangiogenesis. These are correlated to the degree of disease activity. A similar enhancement is seen in the sheath of flexor carpi radialis tendon (*arrow*)

hancement with dynamic sequences after intravenous injection of a paramagnetic contrast agent. It is based on the acquisition of 25 SE T1-weighted sequences at intervals of 15 s from each other, from the beginning of the contrast agent injection (Fig. 59). Subsequently, synovial signal intensity is measured in each scan and is referred to the nearly constant signal intensity given by bone tissue. This results in a curve which has an initial positive trend (rate of early enhancement) and then a plateau (relative enhancement) (Fig. 60). These two parameters, constantly reproducible and not operator dependent, may be used in follow-up studies after treatment.

Another promising technique is kinematic MR (cine-MR) that brings significant advantages in the evaluation of joint function, often heavily limited in RA. A 0.2-T MR unit is used with the "cine" function and a dedicated kinematic tool. This tool enables the keeping of equispaced angular positions, in the range 0° to 50°, of the radiocarpal joint in the movements of flexion-extension and abduction-adduction and their subsequent cyclic visualization to simulate joint movement. Then kinematic reconstructions are performed using GE and SE T1-weighted sequences in coronal and sagittal planes. Kinematic MR accurately shows the normal carpal joint movement and the biomechanical alterations occurring in advanced phases of RA.

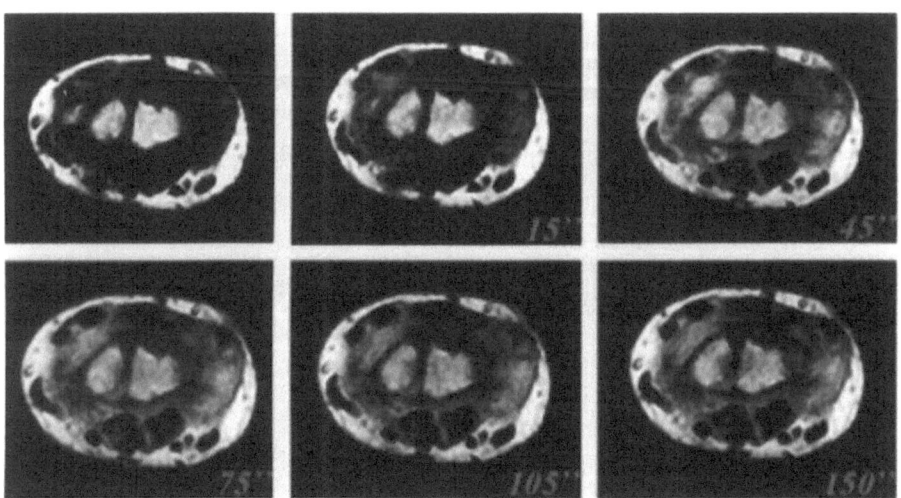

Fig. 59. Dynamic sequences after intravenous insection of contrast agent to evaluate the degree of synovial pannus enhancement

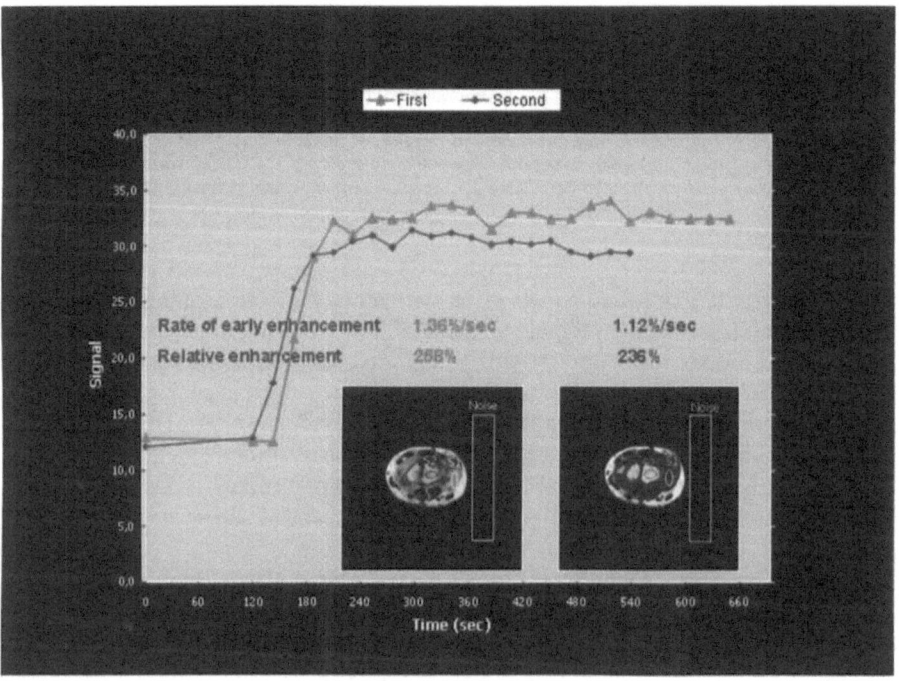

Fig. 60. Curve of the synovial signal intensity measured in each scan after contrast agent injection and referred to the constant signal bone intensity

3 Clinical and Radiological Cases

Inflammatory rheumatic diseases represent an increasing group of diseases which have notable social effects both for the affected patients, whose quality of life decreases, and for the commitment of resources in the medical field. Among these diseases, the most frequent pathology is RA and the hand its most frequently involved localization. Therefore, it is necessary to obtain an accurate evaluation focused, on one hand, on the precise application of the clinical criteria adopted by the American College of Rheumatology, and, on the other hand, on the ever-increasing use of diagnostic imaging which is able to provide essential parameters for the quantification of articular damage.

Taking these points into consideration, we have compiled **25 clinical-radiological case reports** showing the potential of different imaging techniques (conventional radiography, ultrasonography, magnetic resonance) for identifying the different phases of RA.

Each case report, numbered in progressive order but not according to clinical criteria, contains not only radiological documentation but also few anamnestic details. Even if the exact interpretation of a given radiographic picture solves, at least in part, a particular diagnostic problem, it is not always possible to reach a definite diagnosis without being aware of the patient's clinical condition and without the help of a precise clinical-radiological correlation.

This simple case history includes, as well as the patient's *age* and *sex*, a brief *clinical synthesis* with the relative *laboratory tests*.

CASE 1

History

This 35-year-old woman had had RA for 18 months. RA started with metatarsophalangeal involvement, but became rapidly polyarticular. At the time of MRI, she had 12 swollen joints and 25 tender joints and was treated with NSAIDs only. Laboratory tests were as follows: hemoglobin 13.4 g/dl (normal values < 5 mg/dl), ESR 13 mm/h, CRP 11.4 mg/dl, IgM RF 84.4 U, and positive ANA with homogeneous pattern. The patient fulfilled 6/7 ACR criteria for RA.

Imaging

Ultrasonography of the dorsal part of the wrist with transverse scans (**a**) shows synovial fluid effusion (*asterisks*).This area is hypoechoic and contrasts with the hyperechoic bone cortex (*arrowheads*). MR was performed with T1-weighted GE (**b**) and STIR (**c**) sequences. The axial view confirms the synovial fluid effusion seen by US and shows an erosion (*arrow*) of the capitate that was not seen on conventional radiograms.

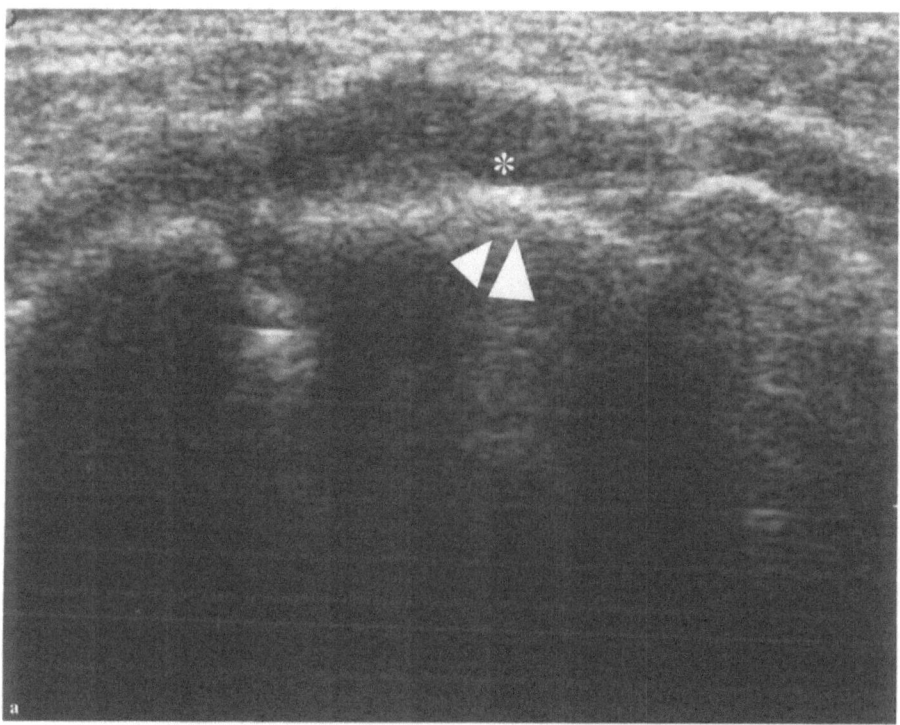

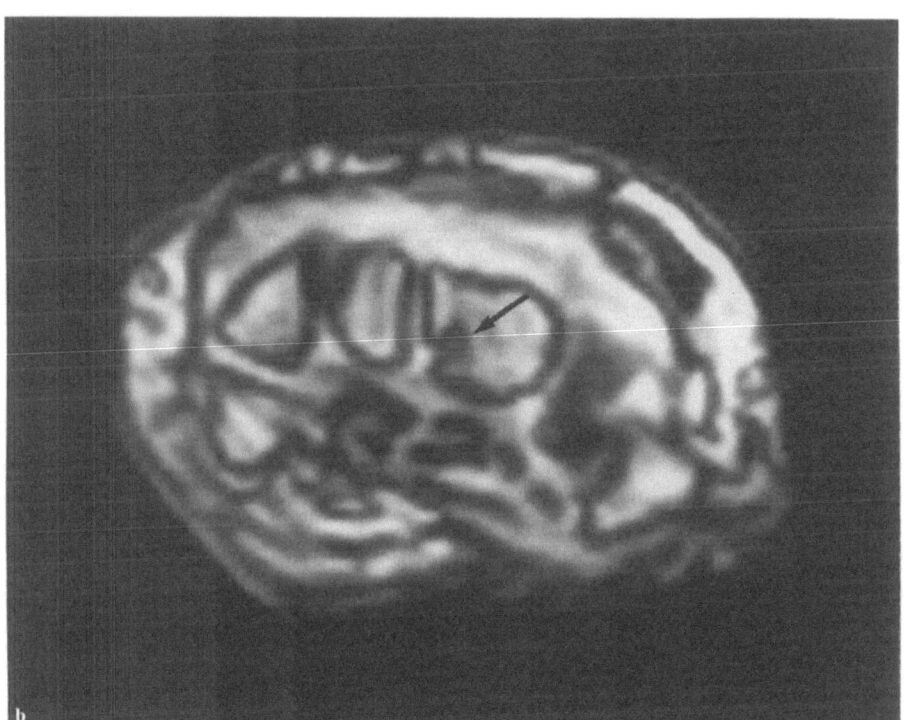

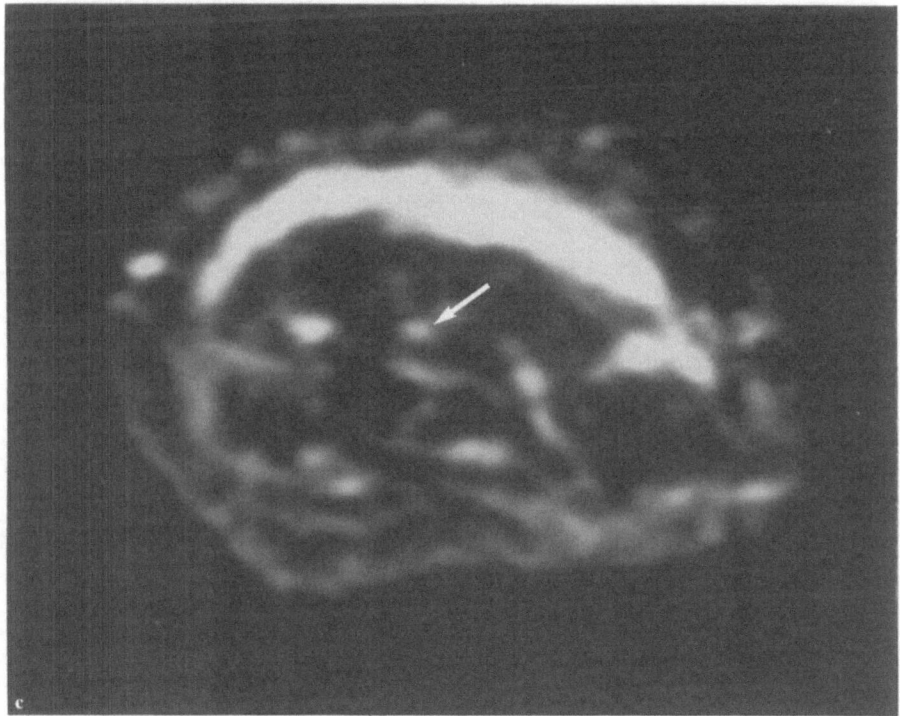

CASE 2

History

Seronegative RA had lasted for 14 years in this 64-year-old woman. At the time of investigation, inflammation of the right wrist was prominent. Her ESR was 15 mm/h, CRP was 7 mg/dl, hemoglobin 12 g/dl.

Imaging

Conventional radiography (**a**) showed joint space narrowing in all the joints of the wrist and several erosions with features of radiolucency. T1-weighted GE (**b**) and STIR (**c**) MR sequences performed in the coronal plane showed a hypertrophic synovial membrane and confirmed the erosive nature of the cystic lesions seen on radiographs. Power Doppler US (**d**) revealed vascular spots, suggesting active synovitis with hyperemia and neoangiogenesis.

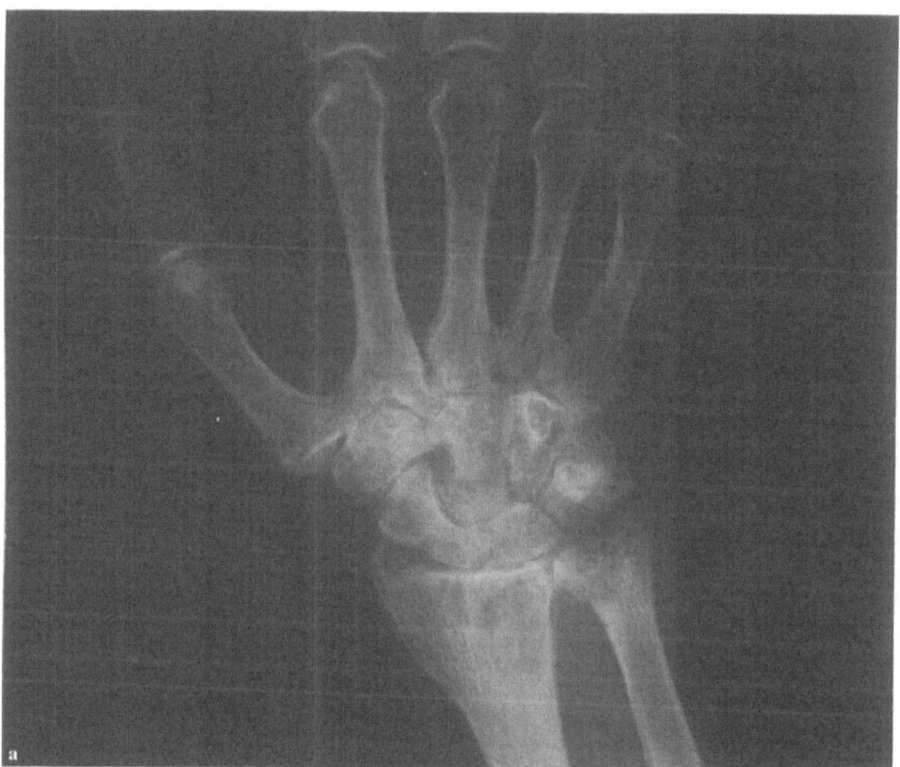

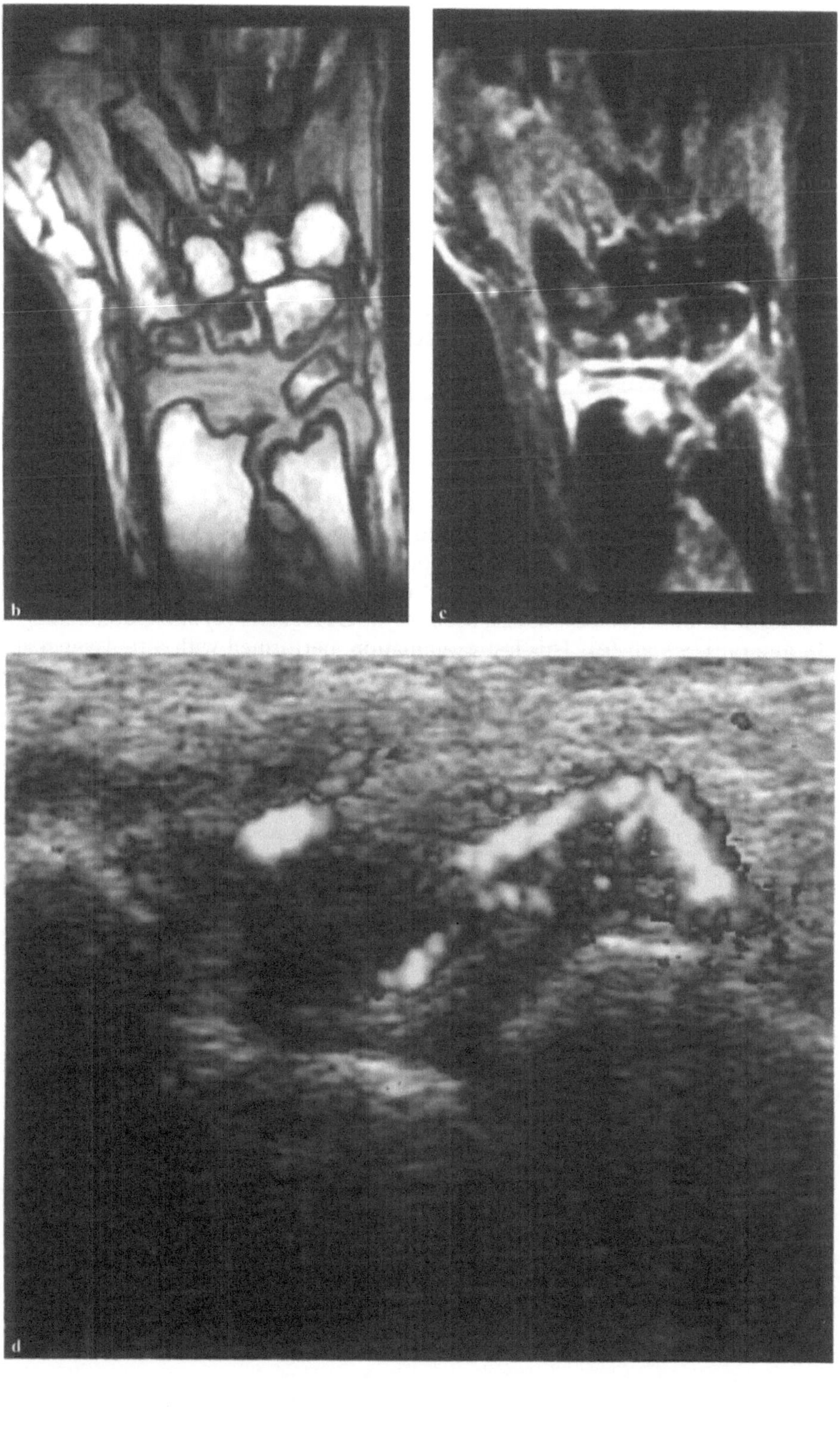

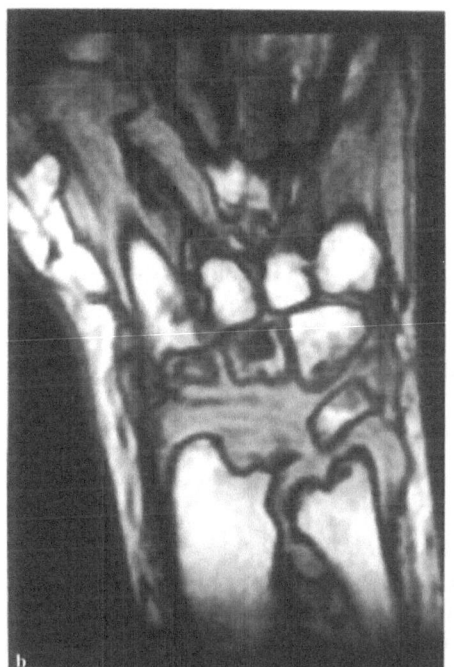
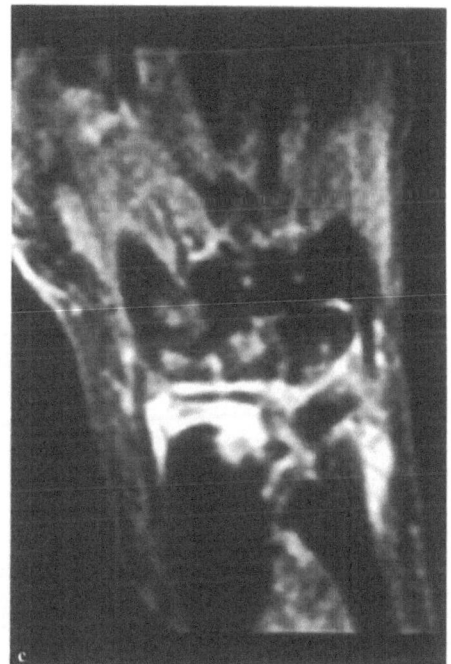

CASE 3

History

A 60-year-old woman had had RA for 7 years. Symmetric polyarticular joint swelling was present with possible involvement of the cervical spine. Frequent periods of remission were achieved with the administration of gold salts and steroids. After stopping gold salts due to poor tolerability, the patient experienced a flare of her disease. At the time of examination, she was relatively well with ESR 20 mm/h, CRP 10 mg/dl, hemoglobin 11 g/dl, and RF 84 U.

Imaging

A posteroanterior radiogram of the hand showed erosions and cystic lesions of the carpal bones, which were partially fused (**a**). The first and third metacarpophalangeal joints were dislocated (**a**). MR confirmed the carpal bone fusion on an axial T1-weighted GE image (**b**). In addition, it showed tenosynovitis of extensor and flexor tendons, which was also seen on the STIR axial (**c**) and coronal images (**d**), and on US scan (**e**). This last examination, performed with a transverse approach on the palmar side of the hand, showed tendon degeneration characterized by fragmentation of the internal fibrillar network.

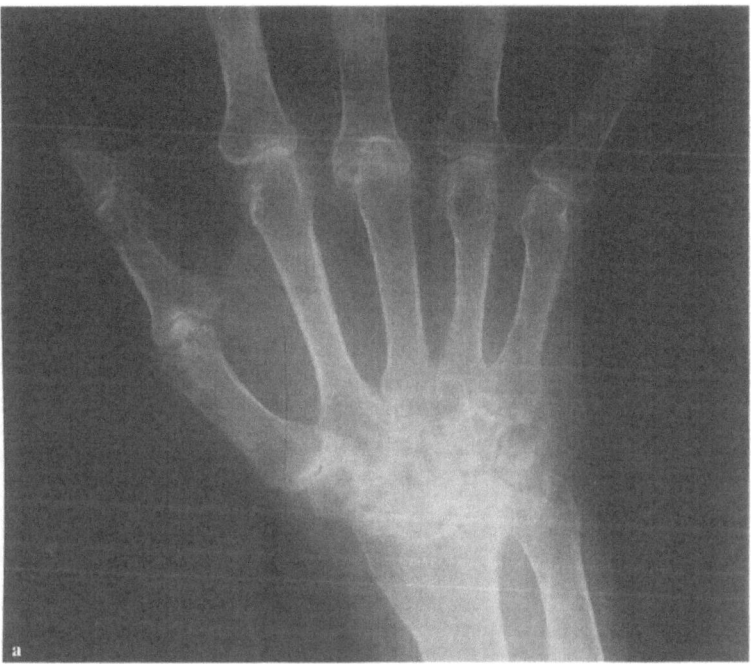

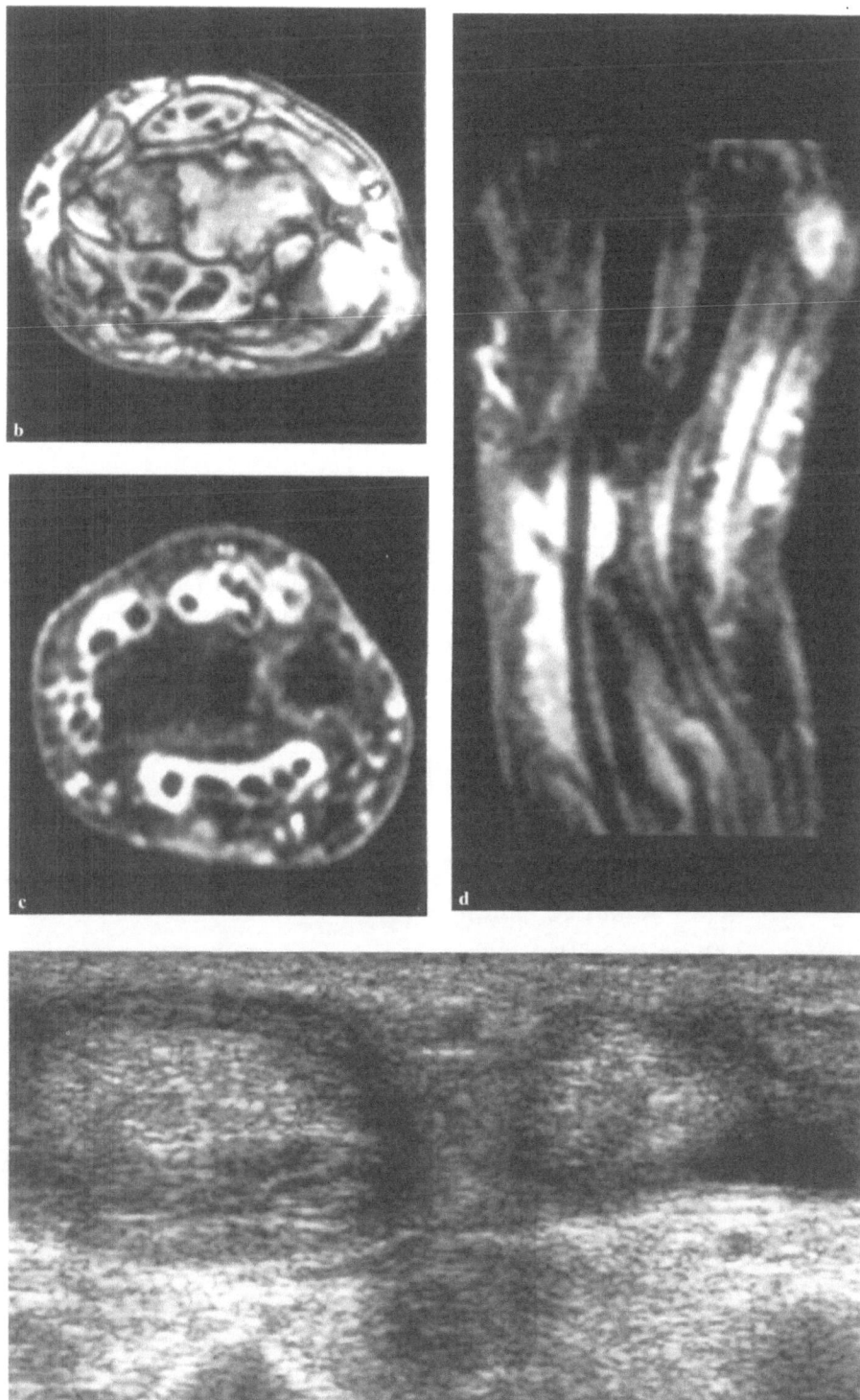

CASE 4

History

RA was diagnosed 11 years previously in this 51-year-old woman. The disease was scarcely erosive and in clinical remission at the time of examination. The pain described by the patient was mainly due to concomitant fibromyalgia. In addition, thyroiditis was present. ESR was 31 mm/h, CRP 4.8 mg/dl, hemoglobin 12.7 g/dl. Treatment was based on oral methotrexate (10 mg weekly), prednisone (10 mg daily), indomethacin (50 mg daily), cyclobenzapride, and paracetamol.

Imaging

A cystic/erosive lesion of the scaphoid is seen on a plain film of the right hand (**a**) (*arrowhead*). This lesion is confirmed by MR performed in the coronal plane with both T1-weighted GE (**b**) (*curved arrow*) and STIR (**c**) (*curved arrow*), as well as by US (**d**) (*arrowhead*). Power Doppler US shows a vascular spot in the synovial membrane infiltrating the erosion (*arrow*).

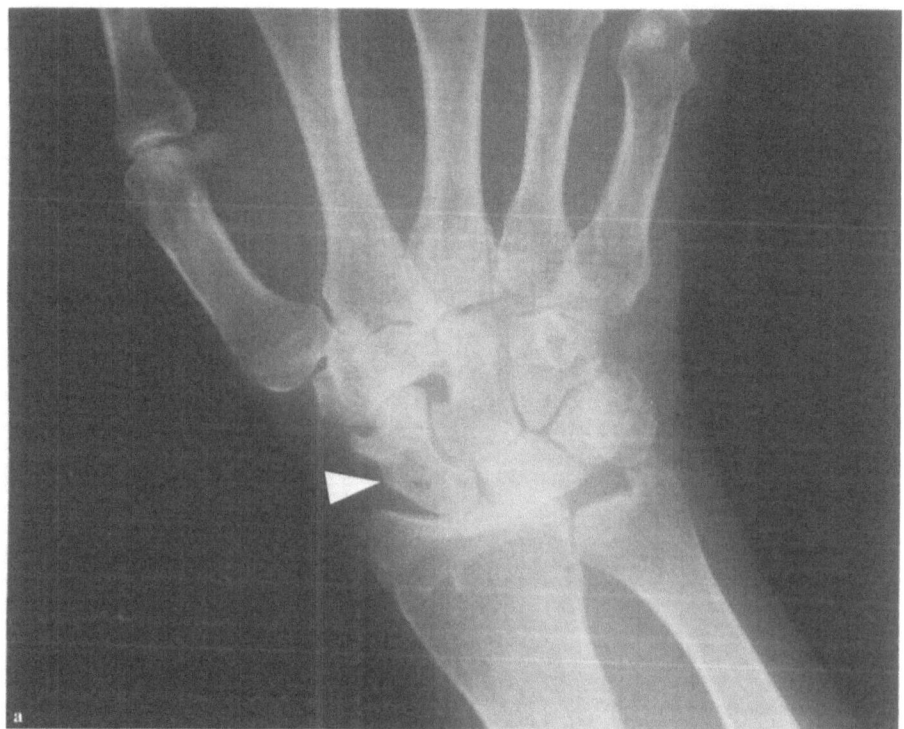

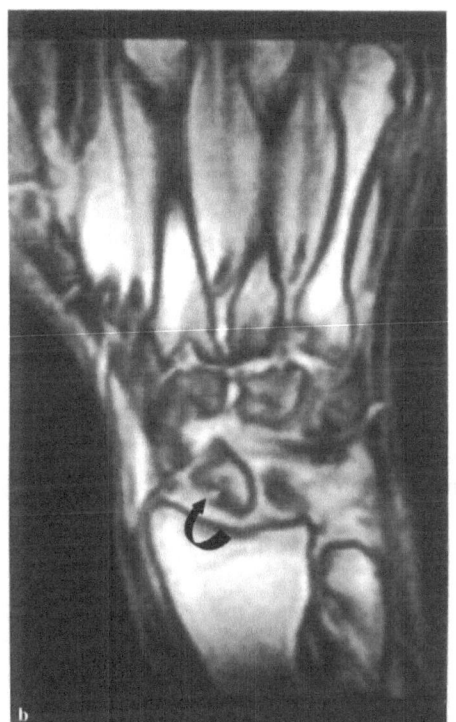
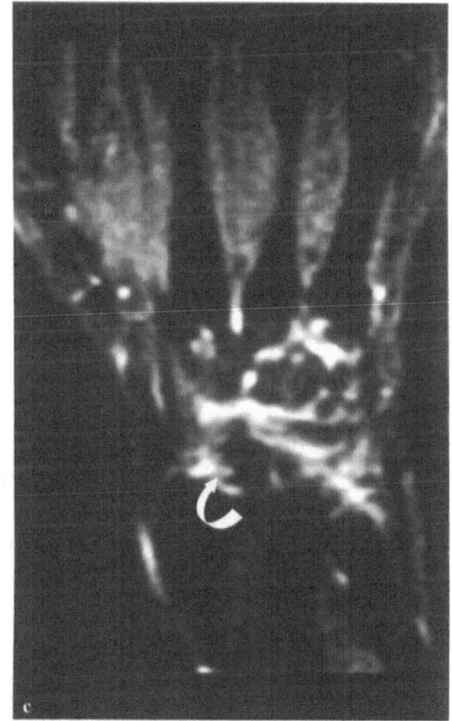
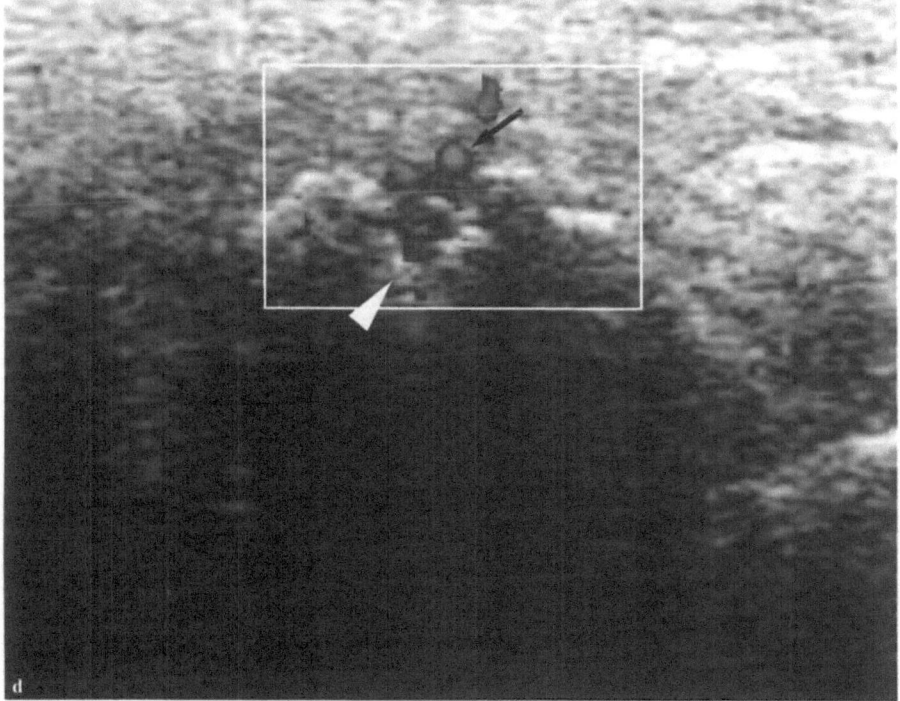

CASE 5

History

This 70-year-old man had had RA for 4 years. The disease mainly affected the hands but was well controlled by therapy. At the time of examination, hemoglobin was 12.8 g/dl, ESR was 10 mm/h, CRP 12 mg/dl, and RF was 198 IU.

Imaging

Plain film of the hand (**a**) shows diffuse osteoporosis, erosive changes, and partial fusion of capitate and trapezoid bones. The fusion is best seen on the coronal and axial GE sequences (**b** and **c**). Synovitis of the ulnar side of the carpus is highlighted by the *arrow*. Note also fragmentation of the triangular fibrocartilage complex.

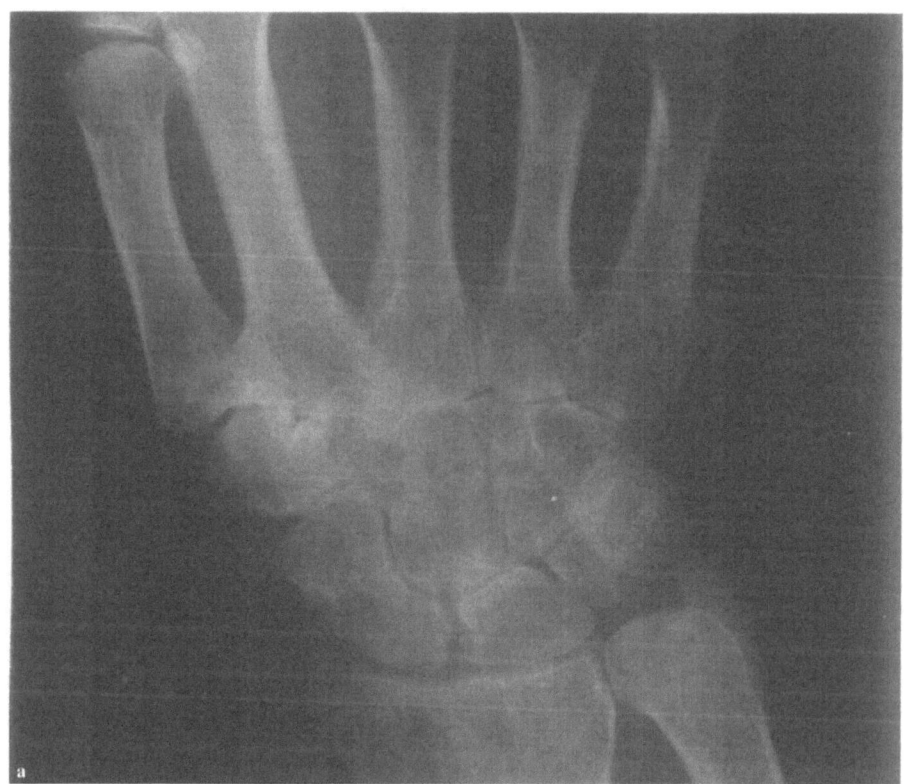

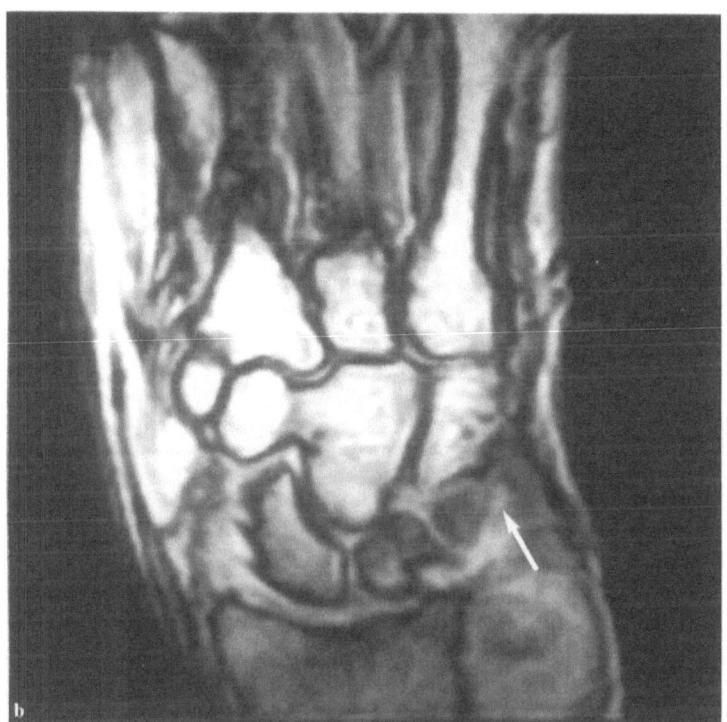

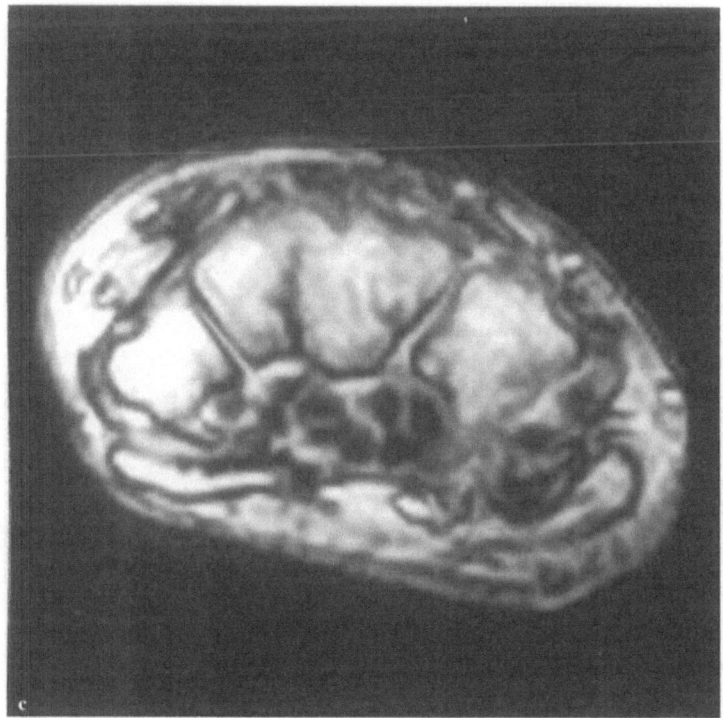

CASE 6

History

Duration of seropositive RA was 4 years when the tests were performed in this 40-year-old man. At the time, the disease was in complete clinical remission with ESR 10 mm/h, CRP 2 mg/dl, hemoglobin 13.6 g/dl. Therapy was based on a combination of methotrexate, sulphasalazine, steroids, and NSAIDs.

Imaging

In accordance with the clinical findings, the radiograph of the hand is substantially normal, with only a radiolucent area of the capitate (**a**). Axial GE T1-weighted (**b**) and STIR (**c**) MRI sequences show minimal tenosynovitis of the extensor digitorum tendon (*arrowheads*) and a large erosion of the capitate corresponding to the radiolucent area seen on the radiograph. A US transverse scan of the distal forearm (**d**) (where the four tendons forming the common extensor of the fingers are close to each other) confirms tendon sheath effusion.

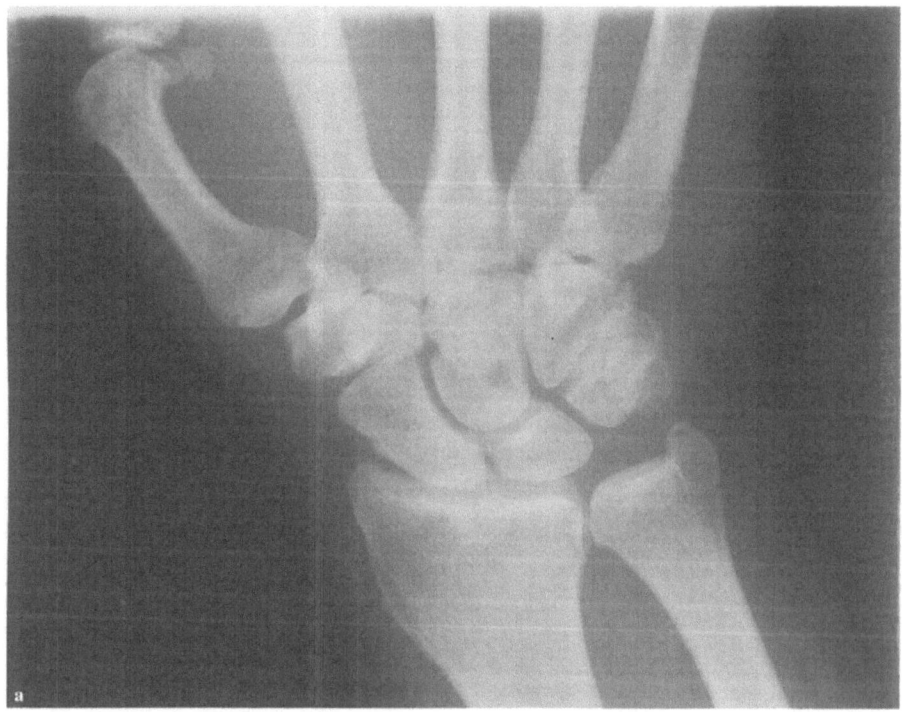

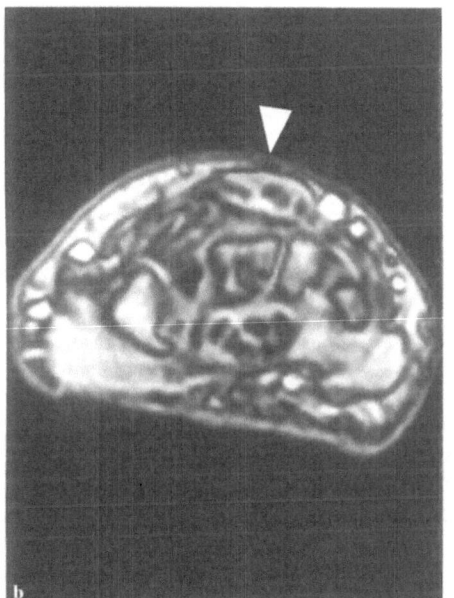
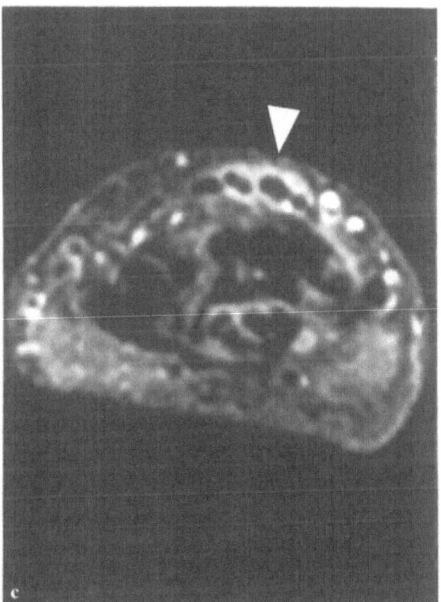

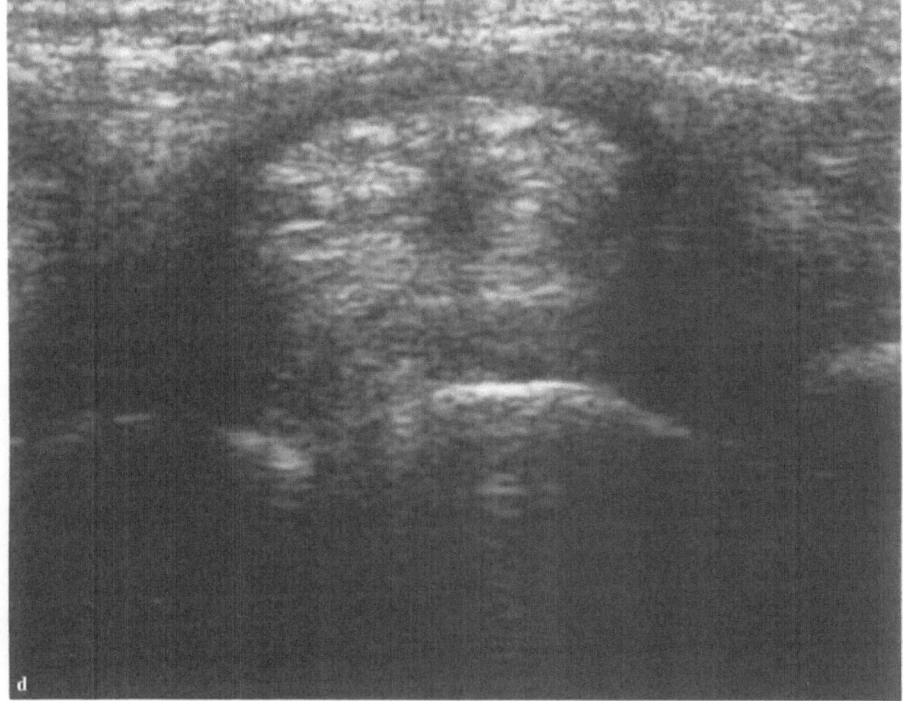

CASE 7

History

This 69-year-old woman had been affected by seronegative RA for the past 8 years. Treatment with methotrexate, steroids, and NSAIDs induced complete clinical remission. At the time of investigation the patient was off therapy and her laboratory tests were as follows: hemoglobin 14.1 g/dl, ESR 11 mm/h, and CRP 2.5 mg/dl.

Imaging

Coronal T1-weighted GE (**a**) and STIR (**b**) sequences show erosions of the distal part of the radius and of the lunate and triquetrum (*arrows*) which are hardly recognizable on plain radiographs (**c**). One erosion is well seen also by a longitudinal US scan on the volar side of the wrist (**d**) (*arrow*). Unfortunately, the absence of clinically active synovitis, did not predict a favorable course. In fact, 5 months after this examination the patient had an acute recurrence of RA.

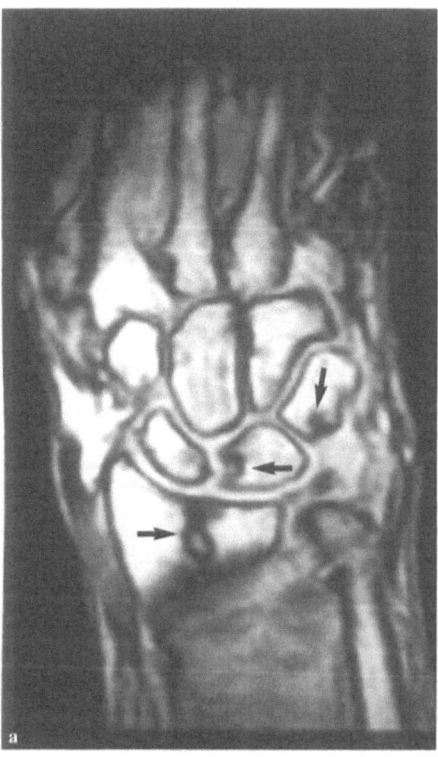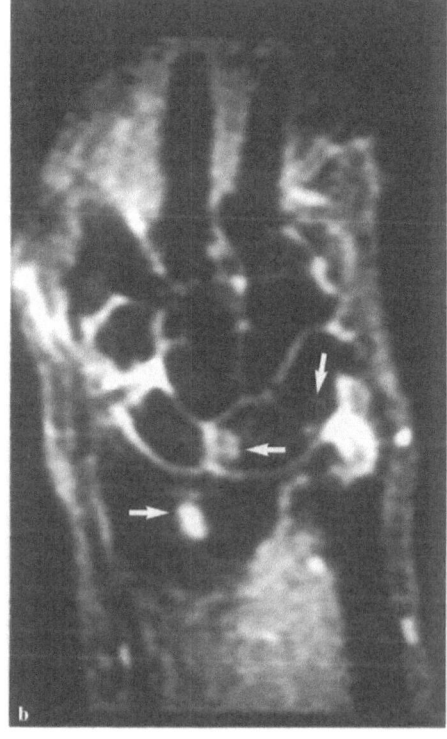

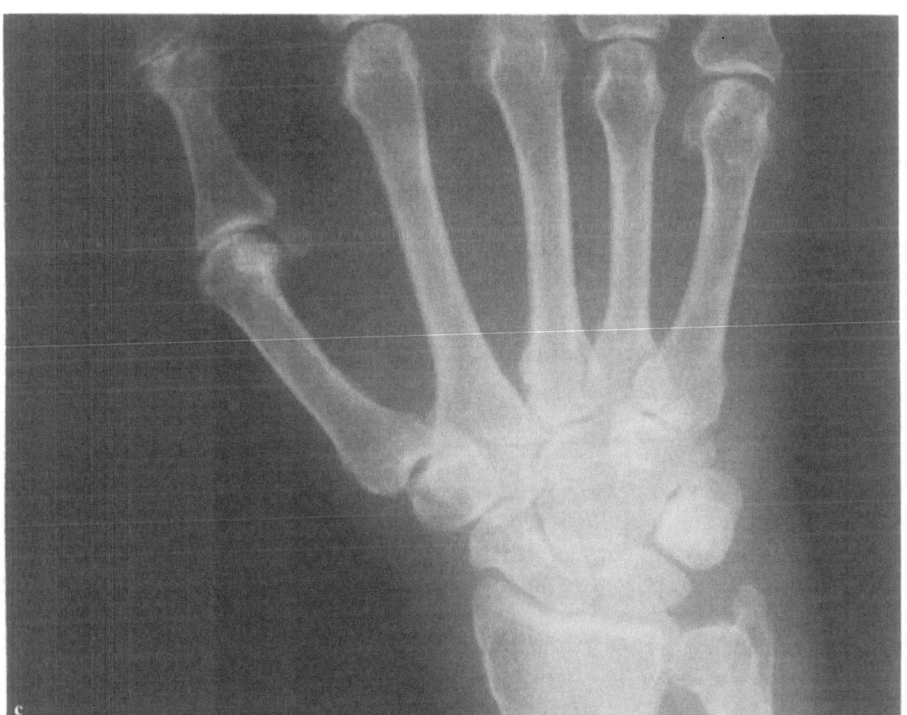

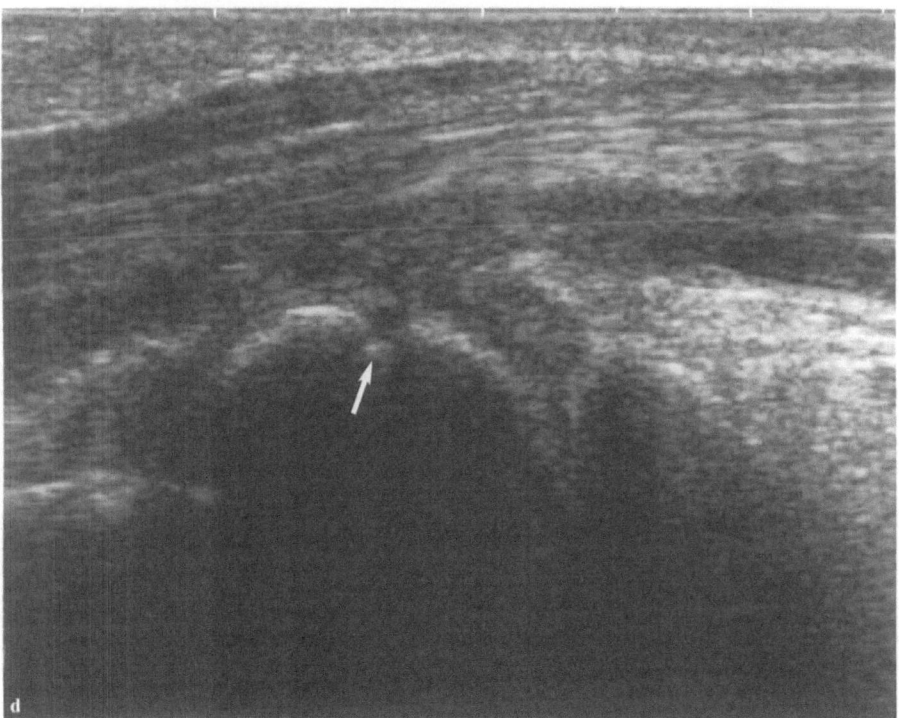

CASE 8

History

The onset of RA in this 70-year-old man had occurred 12 years previously. In the past few years he had been treated with methotrexate and NSAIDs with only fair control of symptoms. In spite of this, laboratory tests improved and at the time of investigation ESR was 8 mm/h, CRP 10 mg/dl, hemoglobin 15.2 g/dl, and RF 133 U.

Imaging

Conventional plain film (**a**) showed osteoporosis, multiple erosions in the wrist and MCP joints, and bony fusion between the capitate and the third metacarpal bone. Axial GE (**b**) and coronal STIR (**c**) MR sequences confirm the presence of erosions and hypertrophic synovial membrane.

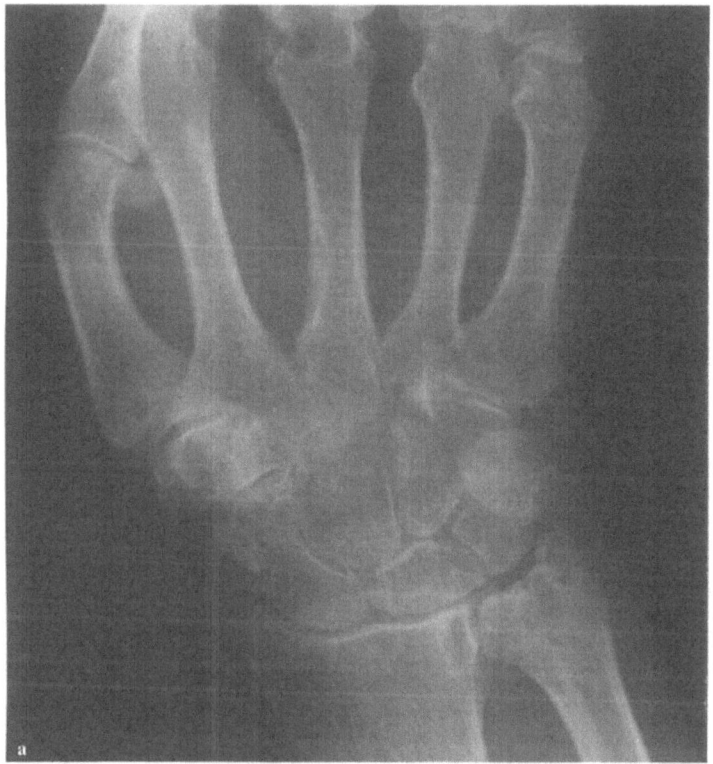

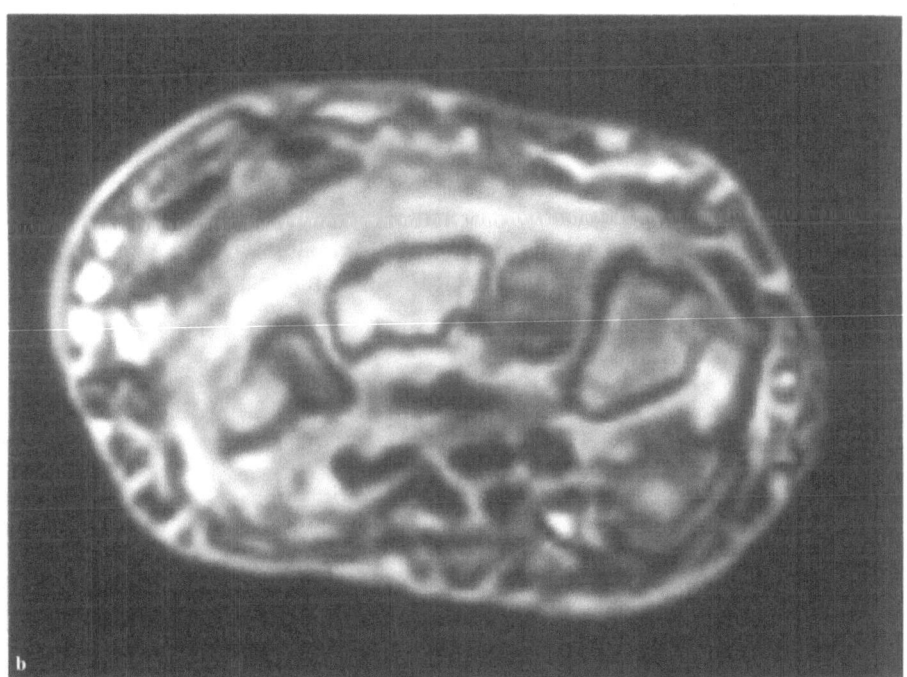

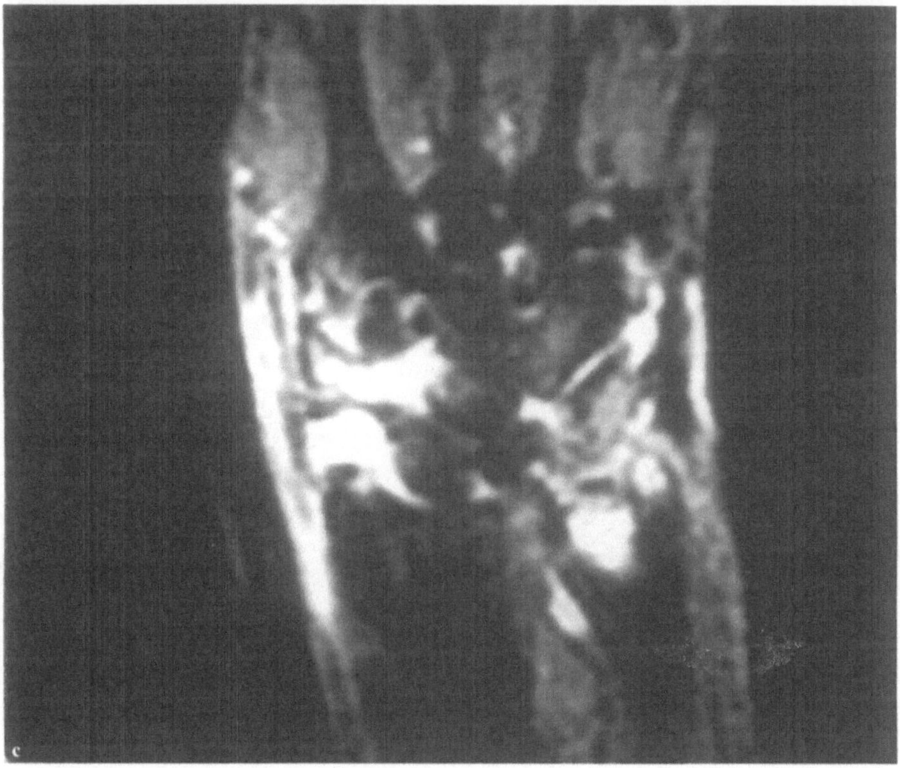

CASE 9

History

This 31-year-old woman with early-onset RA of less than 1 year's duration was admitted to the hospital because of synovitis of the small joints of the hands. At the time of imaging, ESR was 76 mm/h, CRP 16 mg/dl, hemoglobin 10.9 g/dl, and RF 265 U.

Imaging

Radiographs of the hands were normal (**a**), as was the bony component of the wrist on the coronal T1-weighted GE sequence (**b**). In contrast, MRI showed intense synovitis of the radio-ulnar joint on the axial STIR sequence (**c**). Power Doppler US demonstrated that this area is highly vascularized (**d**). Capsular distension of the third and fourth PIP joints is seen on the coronal STIR sequence (**e**).

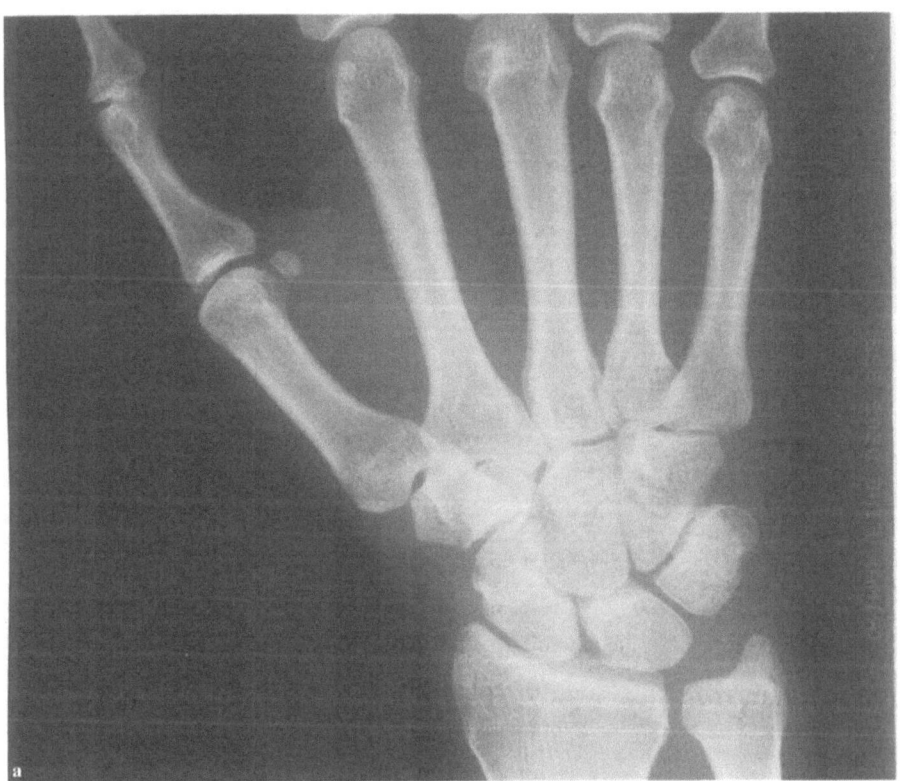

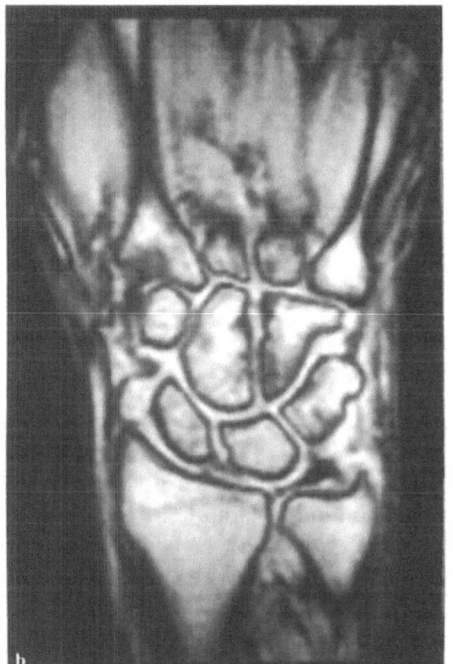

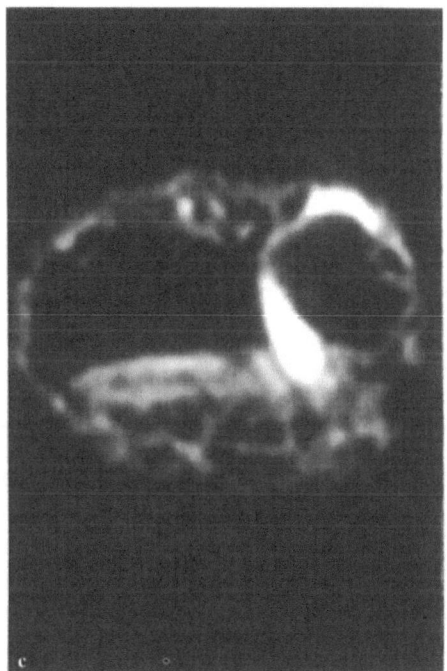

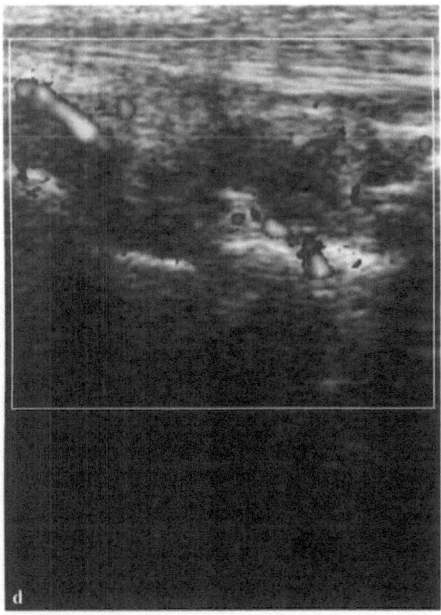

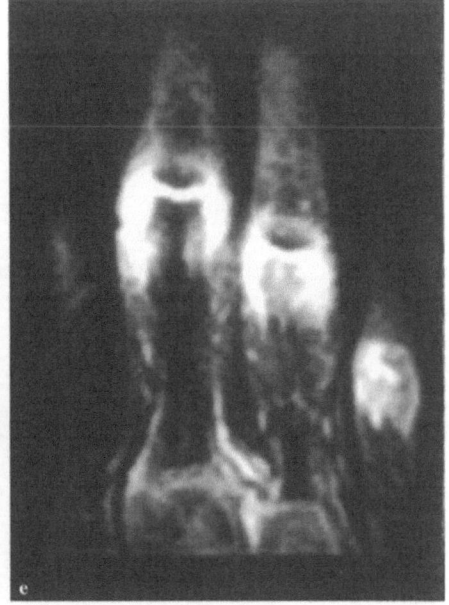

CASE 10

History

The patient, a 59-year-old woman, was diagnosed with RA 8 months before our examination. She had very active disease with hemoglobin 10 g/dl, ESR 75 mm/h, CRP 147 mg/dl, and RF 287 U. Rheumatoid nodules of the elbow were also present.

Imaging

Axial GE T1-weighted (**a**) and STIR (**b**) sequences are more sensitive than conventional radiography (**c**) at detecting bone erosion in the capitate (*arrows*). Note the articular and extraarticular effusions (*curved arrows*). Power Doppler US examination at the same level (**d**) could not give a definite answer to the question of disease activity quantification, because only one vascular spot was present.
MR performed before (**e**) and after the i.v. infusion of paramagnetic c.a. (**f**) shows contrast enhancement in the synovial membrane.

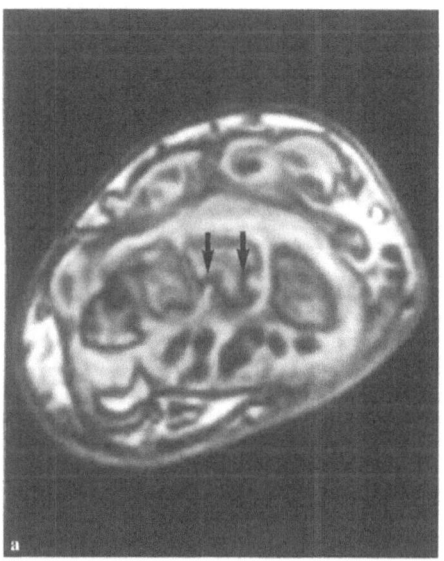
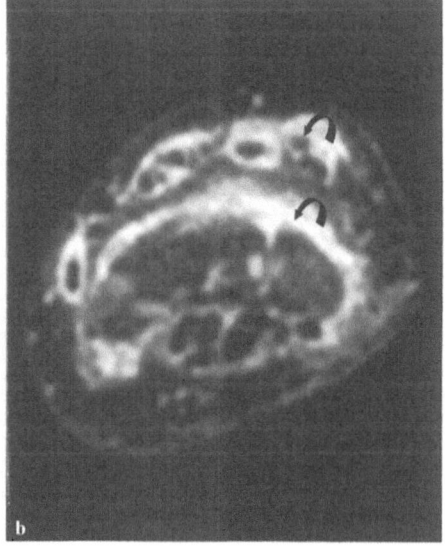

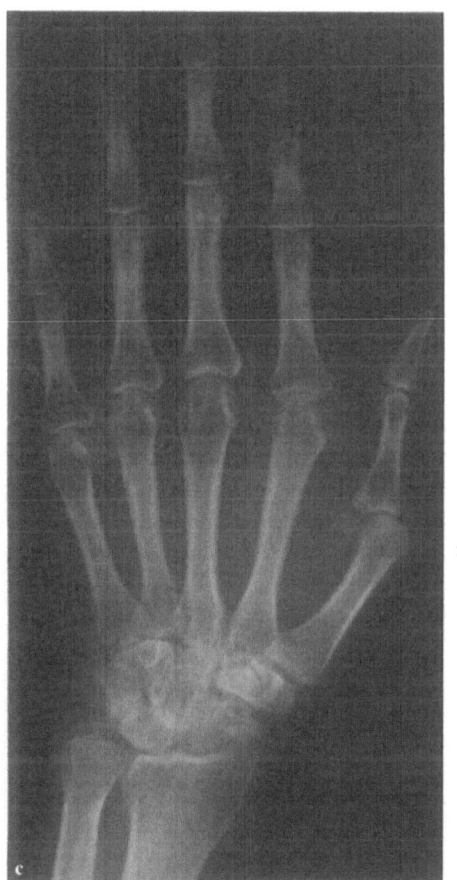

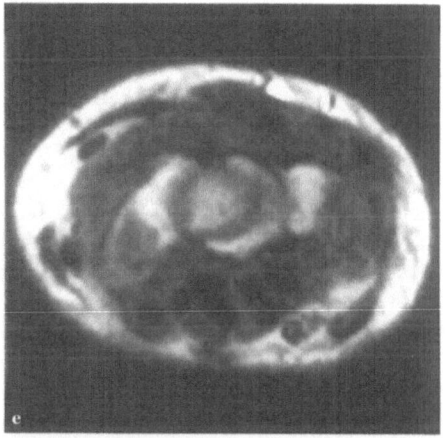

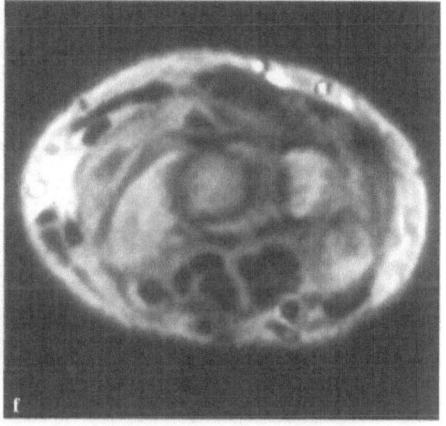

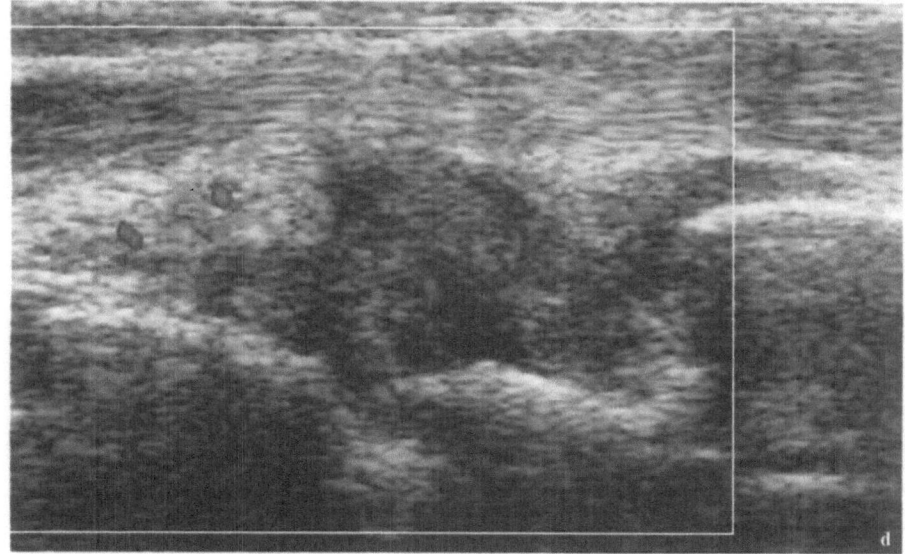

CASE 11

History

After a 10-year course of seronegative RA, this 70-year-old woman still had poly-articular synovitis only partially controlled by steroids and methotrexate. Her hemoglobin was 11.3 g/dl, ESR 40 mm/h, and CRP 51 mg/dl.

Imaging

Conventional radiography (**a**) showed periarticular osteoporosis and a possible cystic lesion of the trapezoid (*arrow*). Coronal GE T1-weighted and STIR images identify the lesion as an erosion (**b, c**). Additional erosions can be seen at the base of the second metacarpal (*arrows*). Axial and sagittal STIR images show synovial effusion in the flexor tendon sheath of the fifth finger (**d, e**). US confirms tenosynovitis of the fifth finger (**f**) with a normal internal echotexture.

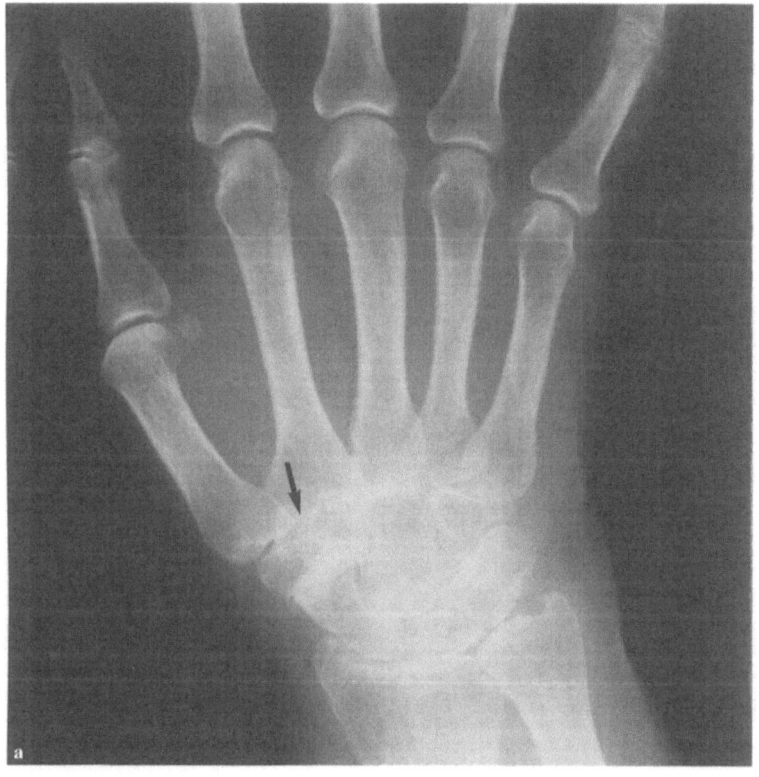

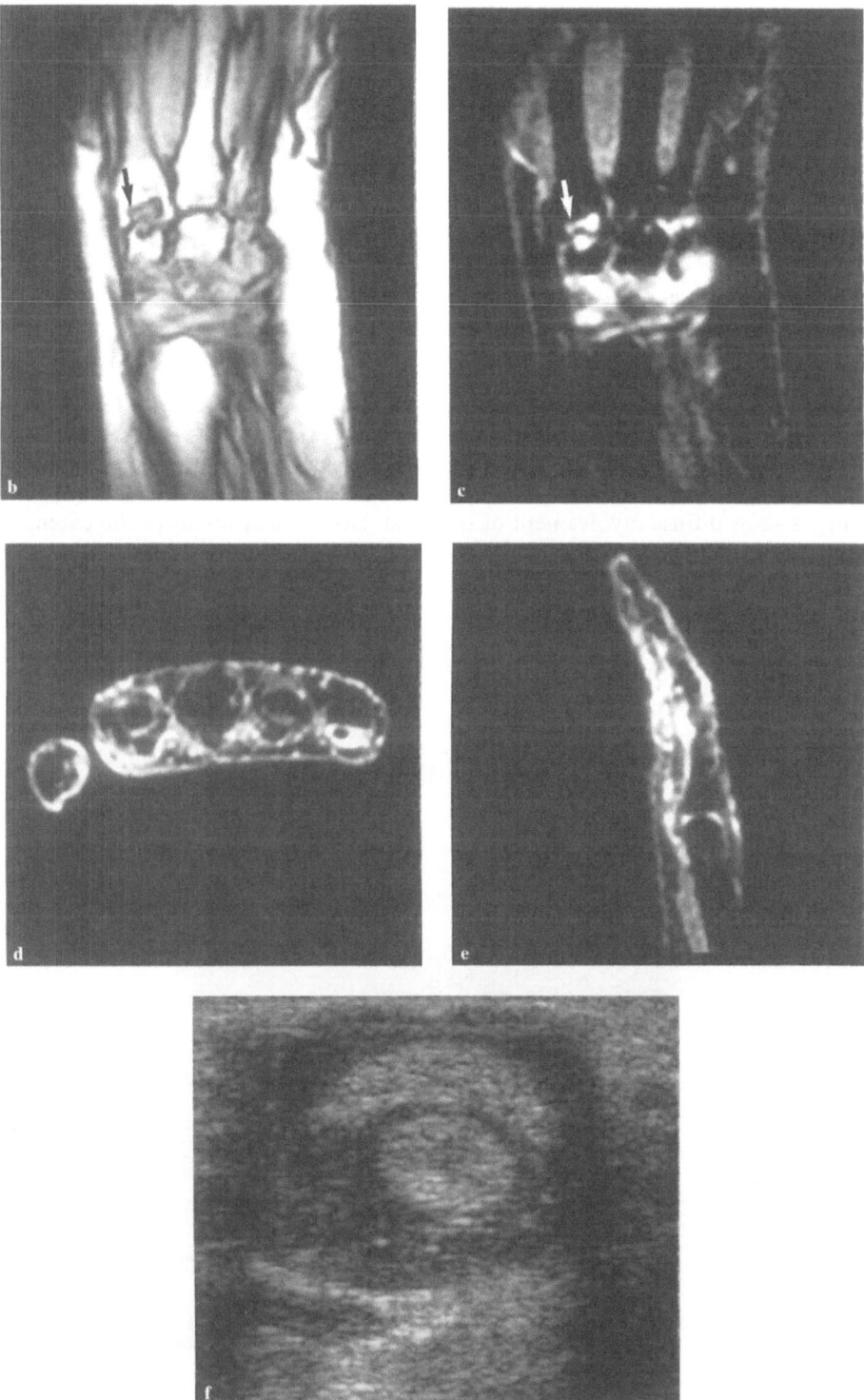

CASE 12

History

This 62-year-old man was affected by seronegative RA which had started about 5 years previously with carpal tunnel syndrome. At the time of examination his hemoglobin was 12 g/dl, ESR 66 mm/h, and CRP 5.3 mg/dl. Rheumatoid nodules were present at the finger tips, despite the absence of IgM rheumatoid factor.

Imaging

Coronal GE T1-weighted (a) and STIR (b) MR images show fluid and synovial inflammatory tissue of the PIP joint. Axial GE T1-weighted (c) and STIR (d) MR images show diffuse involvement of the wrist. Note tenosynovitis of the extensor carpi ulnaris tendon (*arrow*).

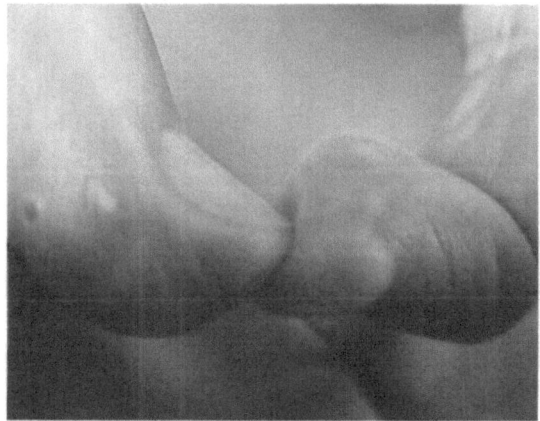

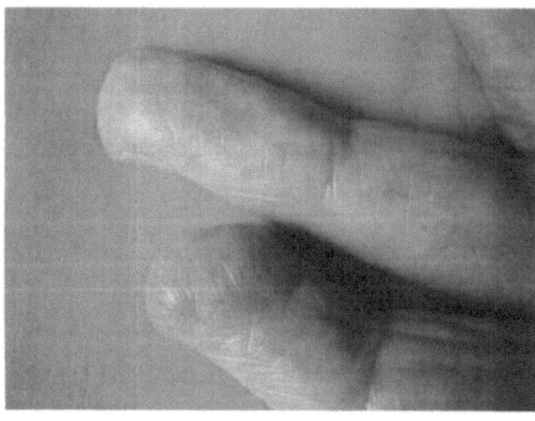

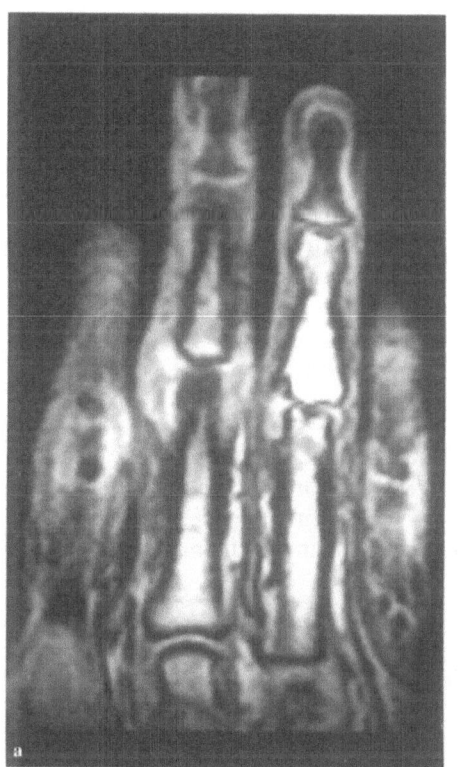

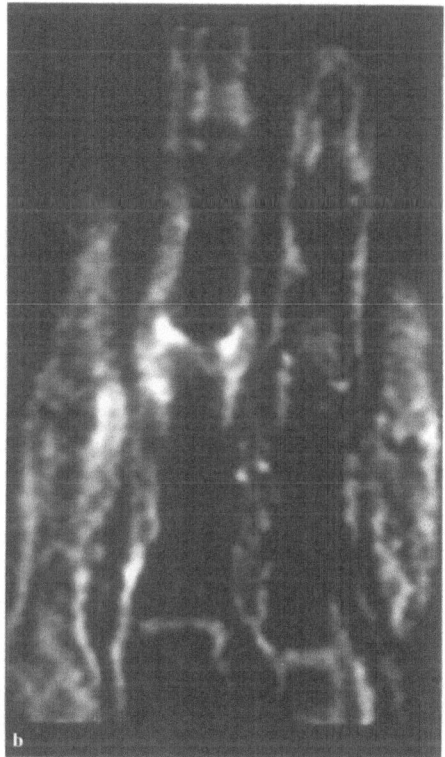

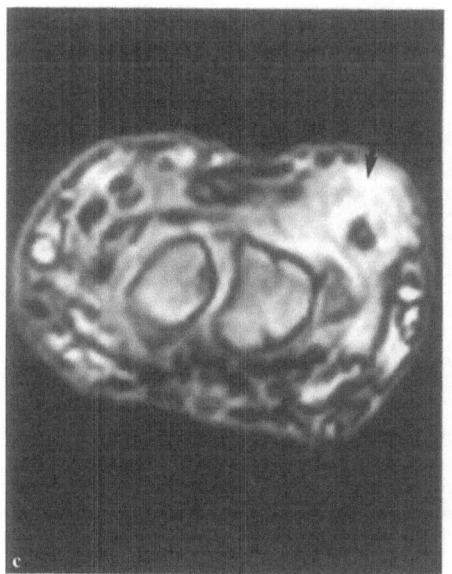

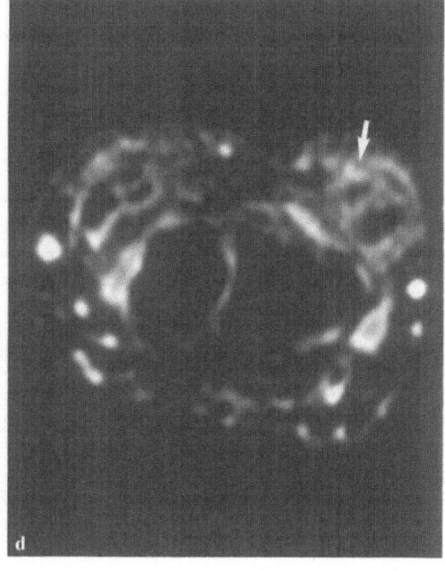

CASE 13

History

This is the same patient as case 12, a 62-year-old man affected by seronegative RA which had started about 5 years previously with carpal tunnel syndrome. At the time of examination his hemoglobin was 12 g/dl, ESR 66 mm/h, and CRP 5.3 mg/dl.

Imaging

An erosion of the first metacarpal head is seen on the plain film of the hand (**a**) where also soft-tissue swelling is present (*arrow*). Coronal GE T1-weighted (**b**) and STIR (**c**) MR images confirm the erosion of the first metacarpal (*arrow*). US evaluation performed with a 20-MHz (**d**) transducer shows the bone changes and the synovial effusion.

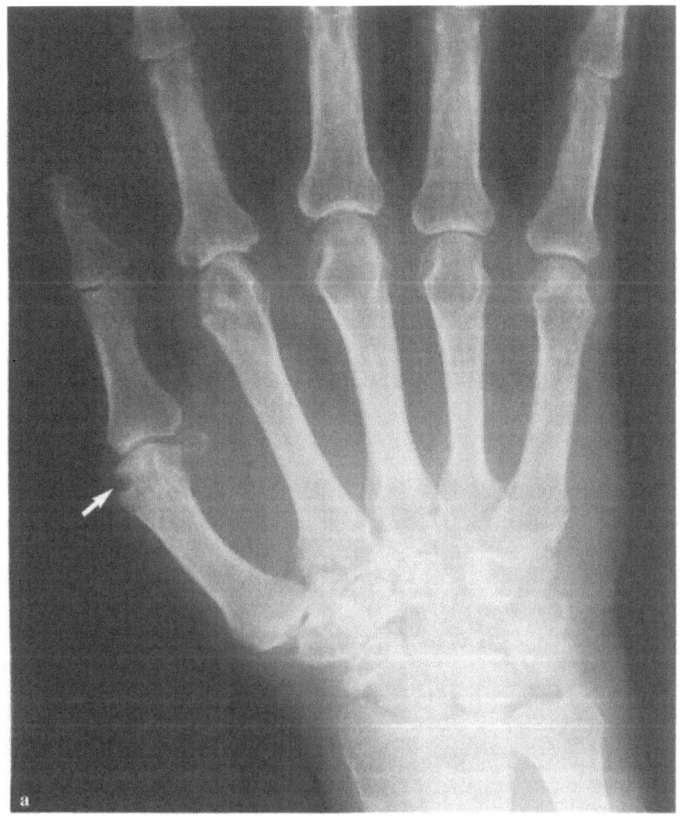

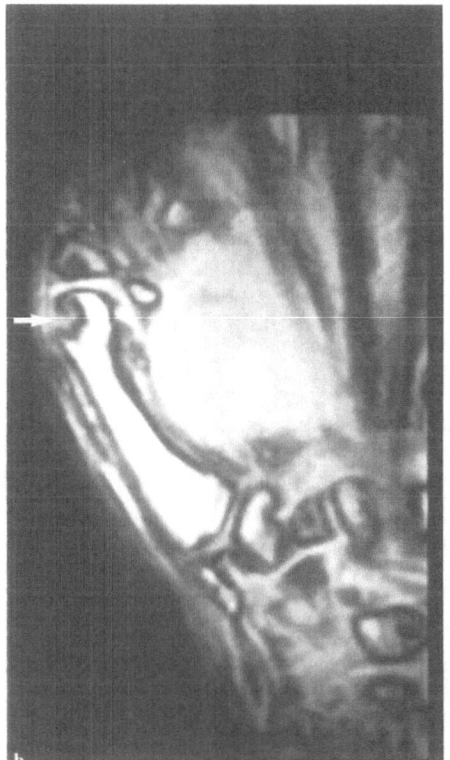

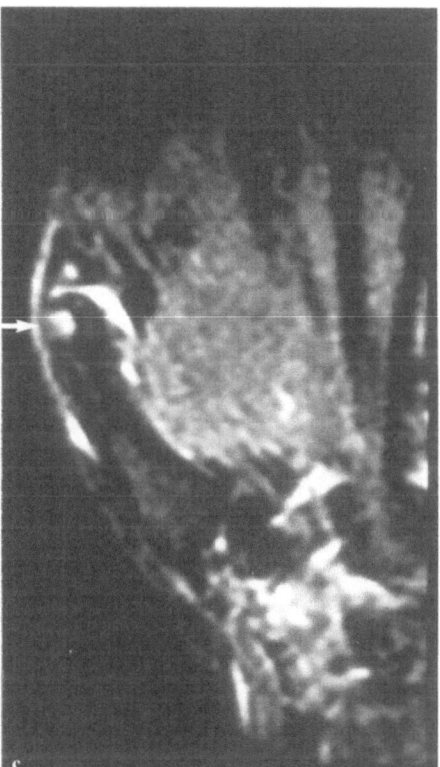

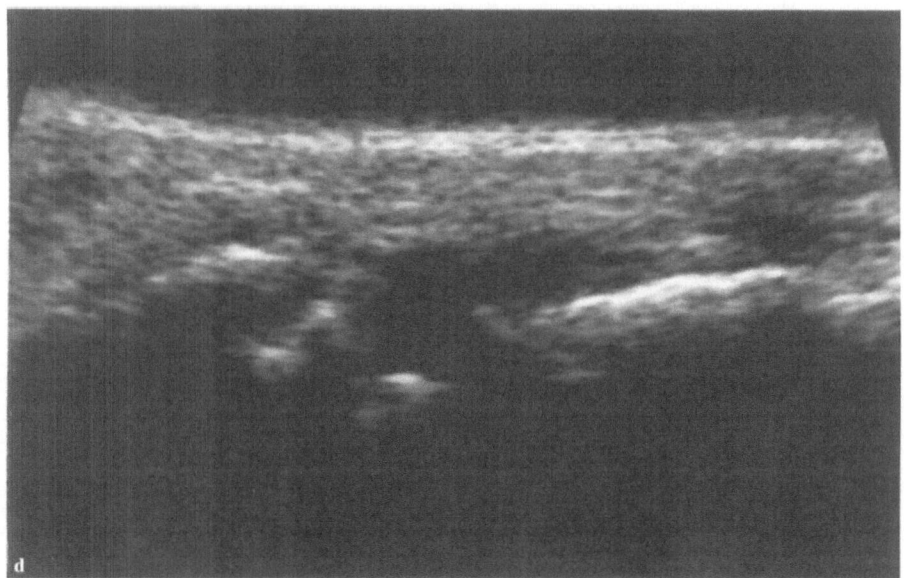

CASE 14

History

Seronegative RA, associated with allergic dermatitis and bronchiectasia, had affected this 46-year-old woman for the previous 9 years. Hemoglobin was 13.7 g/dl, ESR 42 mm/h, and CRP 28 mg/dl.

Imaging

Conventional radiography shows joint space narrowing, erosions, and cysts of the wrist bones and the head of the ulna as well as scapho-lunate ankylosis (**a**). Axial MR with T1-weighted GE (**b**) and STIR (**c**) sequences shows tenosynovitis of the common extensor tendon. This finding is well seen by US (**d**).

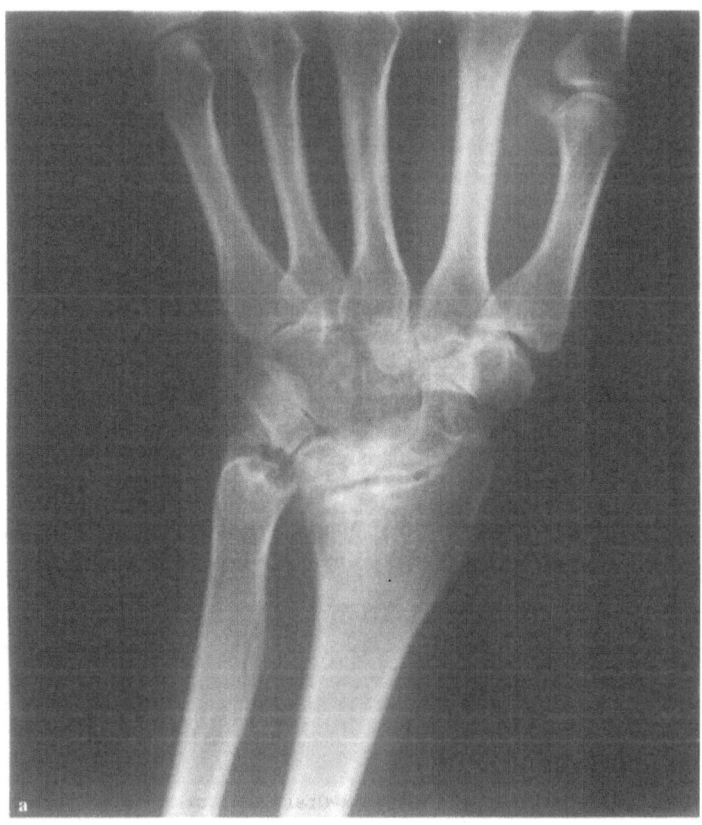

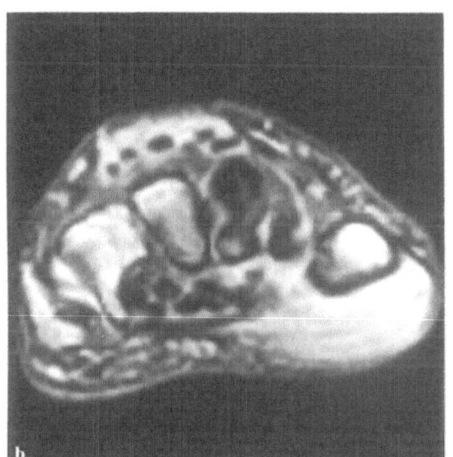
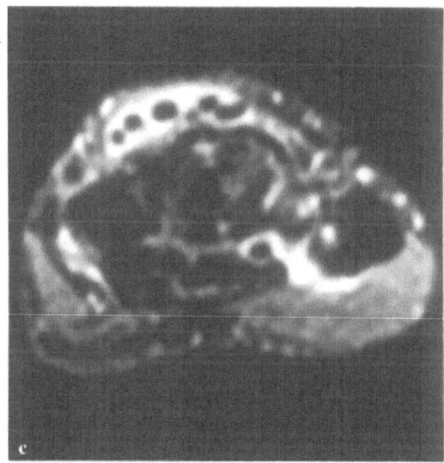

IST.RADIOLOGIA DIMI GENOVA   27 SET 00   15:54

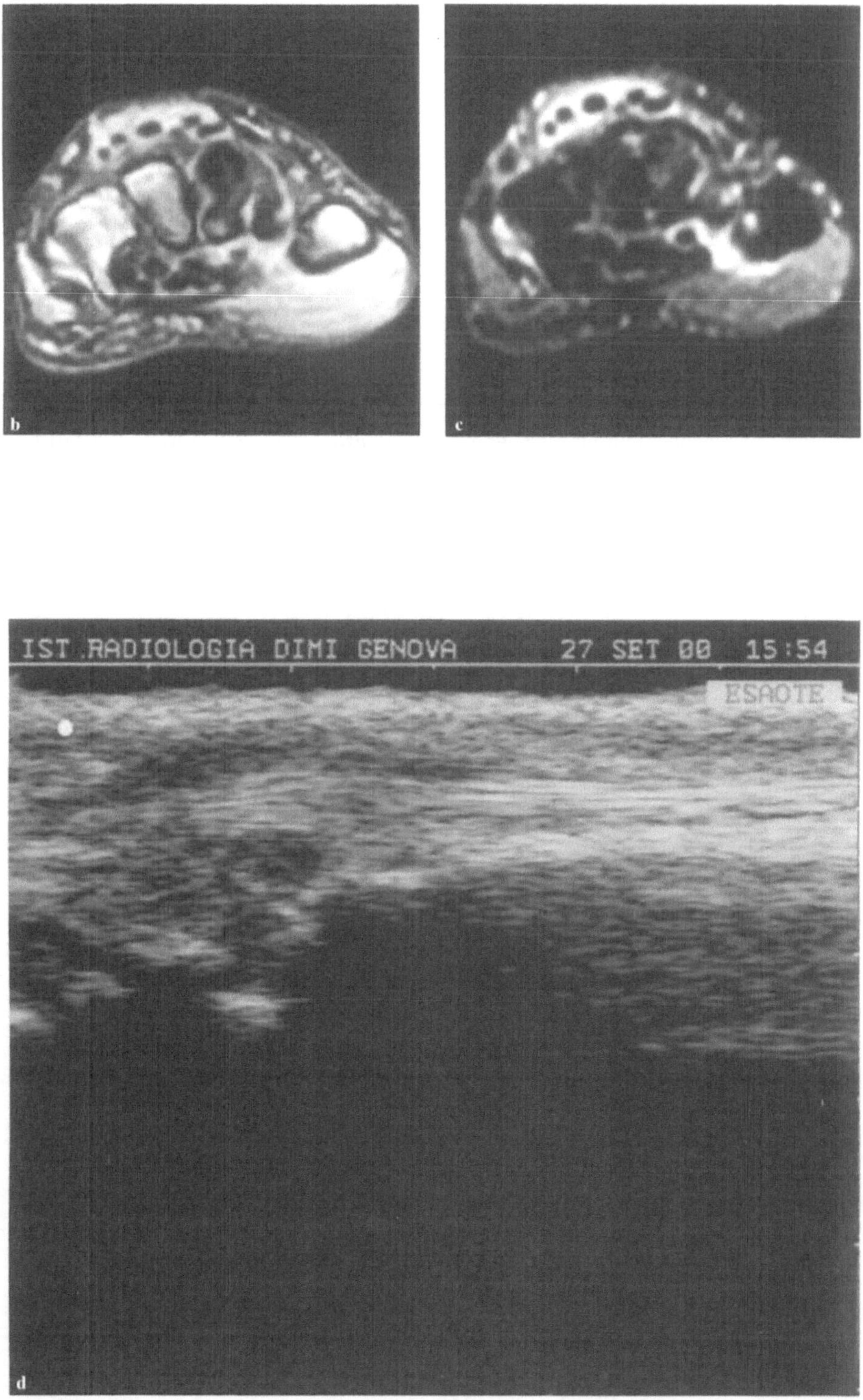

CASE 15

History

This 72-year-old man had had mild RA for 5 years. Hemoglobin was 12.3 g/dl, ESR 40 mm/h, CRP 3 mg/dl, and RF 100 U.

Imaging

Coronal MR with T1-weighted GE and STIR sequences shows an erosion of the hamate which is hypointense on the GE (**a**) and hyperintense on the STIR (**b**) sequence. This aspect can be also seen on conventional radiography (**c**). Additional findings are synovial effusion on the radial side of the wrist (*asterisk*) and disruption of the triangular fibrocartilage (*arrowhead*). A longitudinal Power Doppler scan performed on the dorsal side of the radiocarpal joint confirms the effusion. In addition, vascular spots are seen in the inflamed synovial proliferation (**d**).

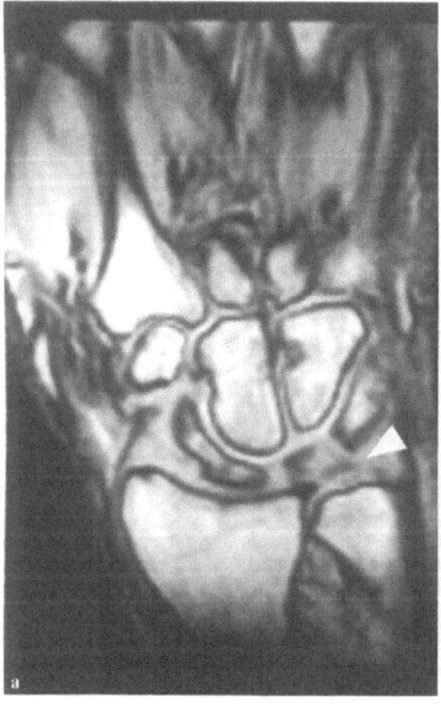
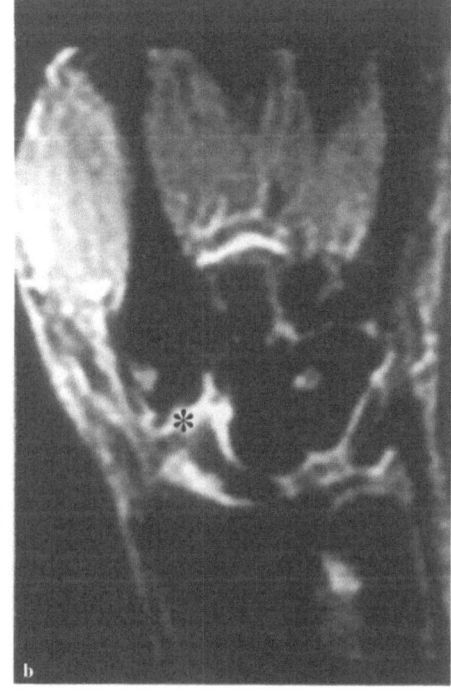

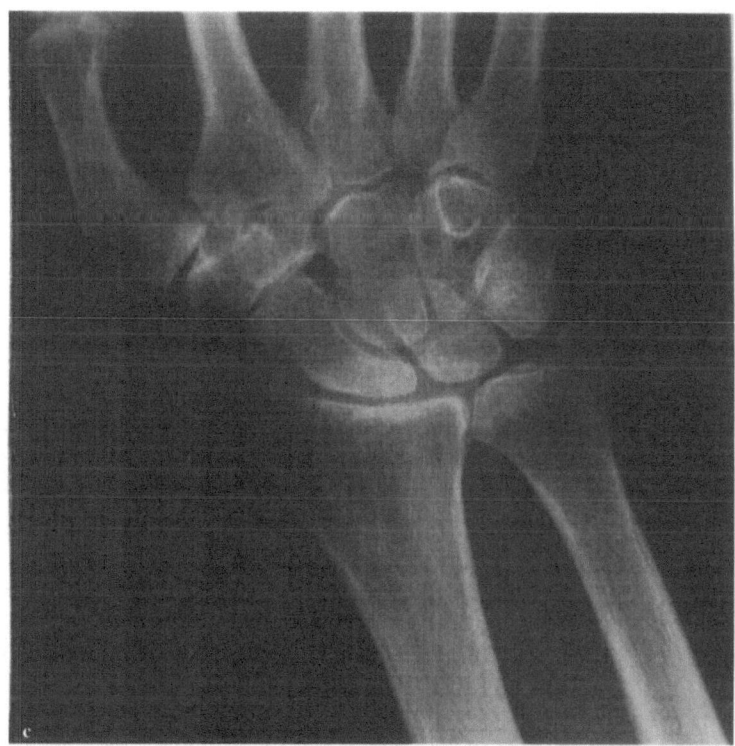

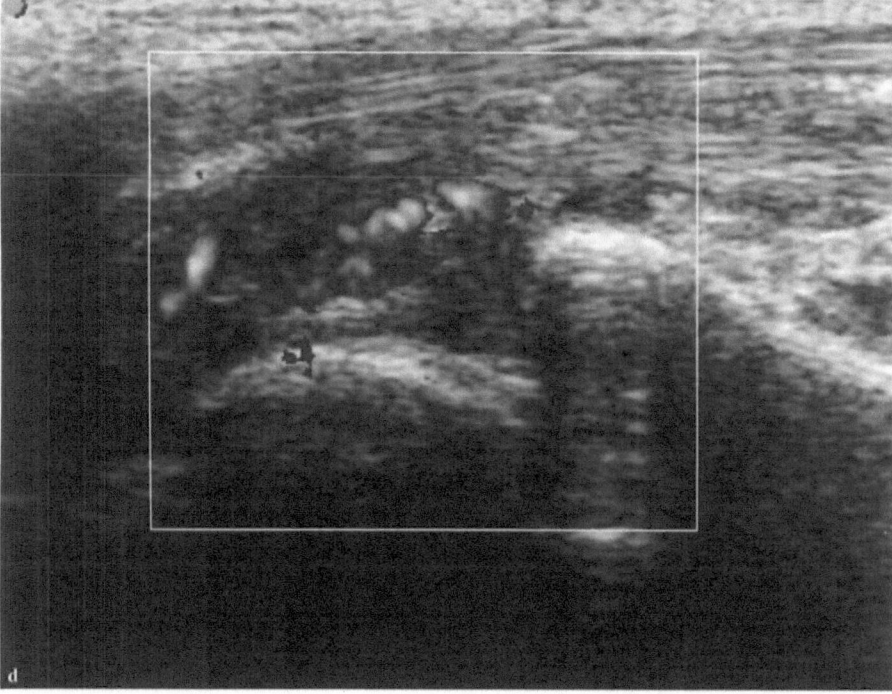

CASE 16

History

In this 71-year-old woman, seropositive RA had been diagnosed 8 years previously. She also showed rheumatoid nodules and scleromalacia. Her hemoglobin was 10.3 g/dl, ESR 120 mm/h, and CRP 55.6 mg/dl.

Imaging

Axial T1-weighted GE (**b**) and STIR (**c**) sequences show an evident erosion of the distal radius. There is also synovial hypertrophy and fluid effusion around the ulnar styloid. This synovial involvement is clearly shown by US examination (**a**). Power Doppler US allows evaluation of disease activity through demonstration of increased vascular flow.

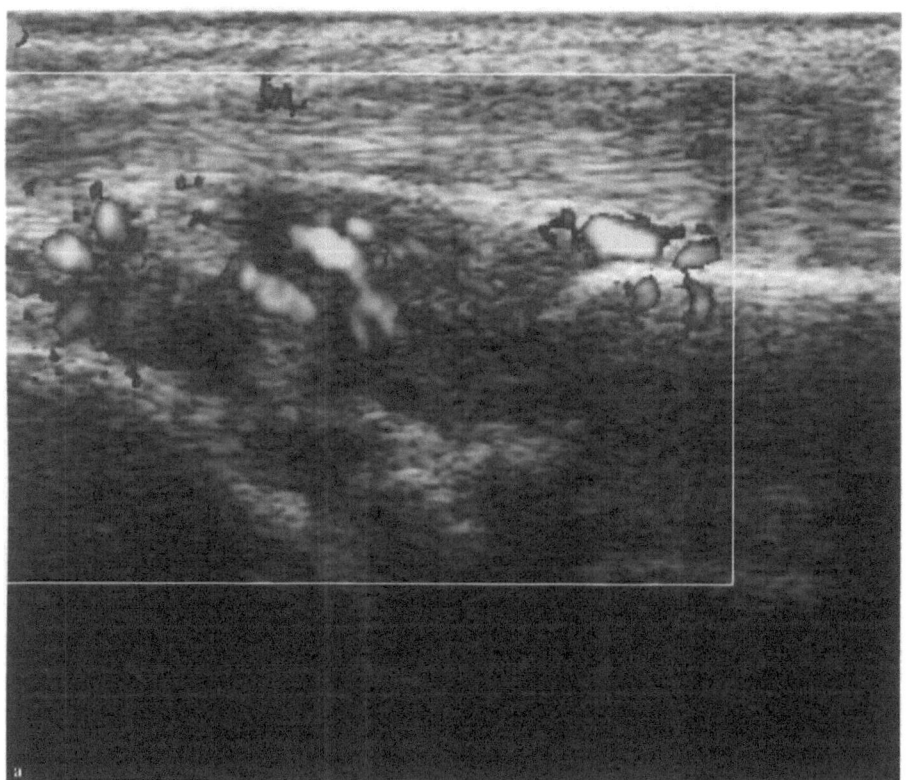

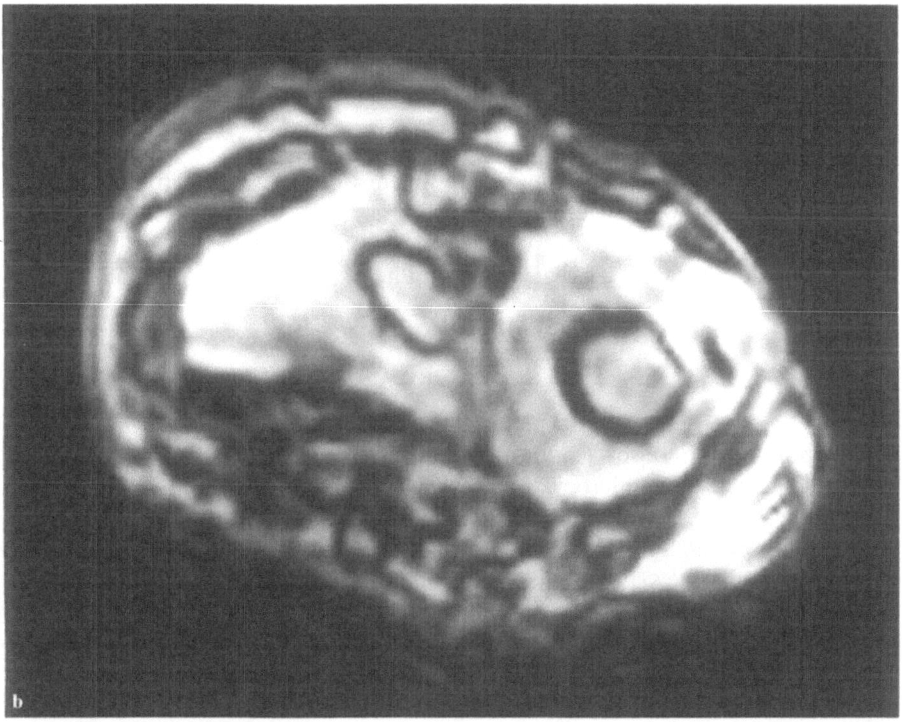

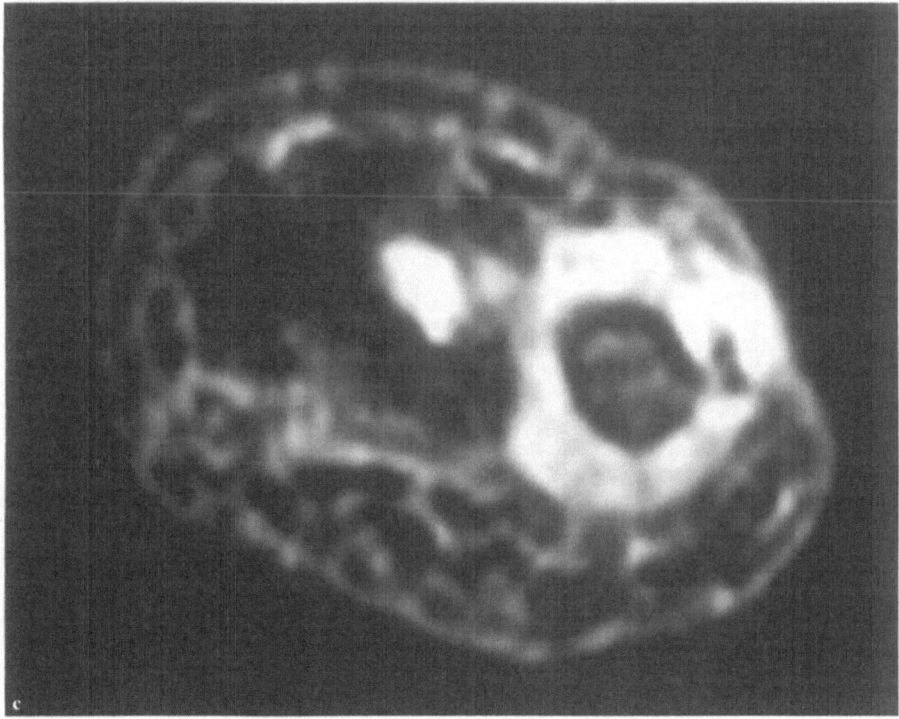

CASE 17

History

This patient is a 54-year-old woman with recent-onset RA of 6 months' duration. Her PIP joints and wrists were swollen, with associated carpal tunnel syndrome. The disease was apparently controlled by an association of methotrexate and gold salts. Hemoglobin was 13.6 g/dl, ESR 18 mm/h, and CRP 1.2 mg/dl.

Imaging

Conventional radiography (**a**) shows involvement of the first carpo-metacarpal joint and multiple bone microcysts on several wrist bones. An axial STIR sequence (**b**) demonstrates synovial inflammation in the periulnar compartment and intense tenosynovitis of the flexor tendons. Coronal GE T1-weighted and STIR (**c, d**) sequences demonstrate synovial fluid effusion in the PIP joints of the second, third, fourth, and fifth fingers. Note also a large erosion of the head of the third metacarpal bone. Power Doppler US (**e**) demonstrates marked tenosynovitis, hyperemia and new blood vessel formation in the synovial proliferation.

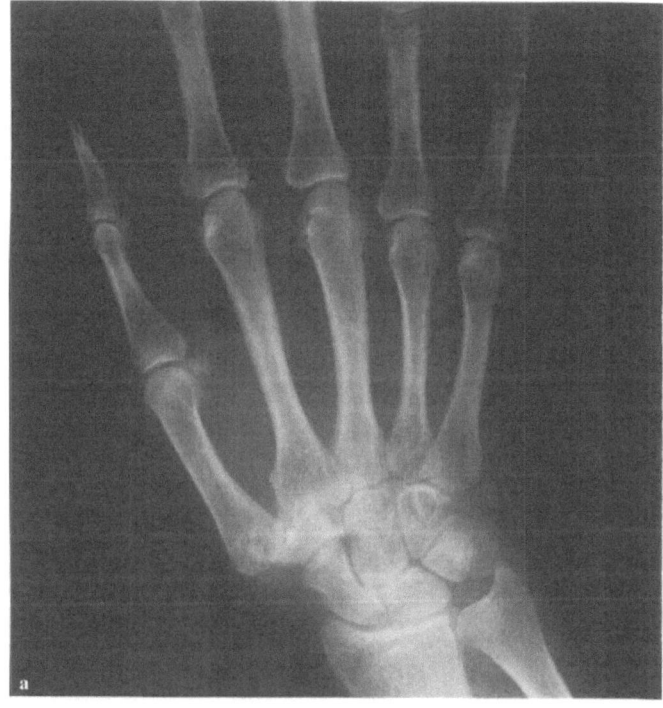

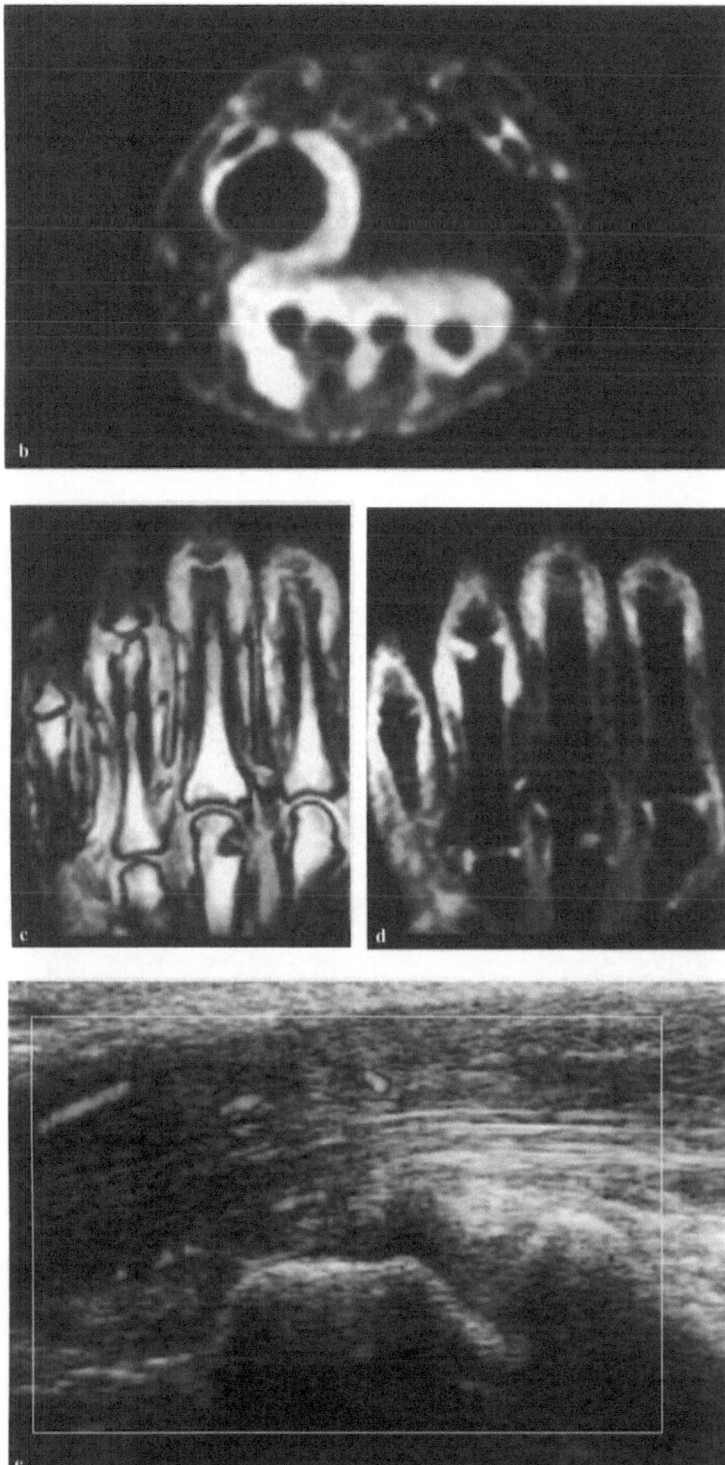

CASE 18

History

This 40-year-old woman had been affected by RA since age 28. The disease was active with hemoglobin 11 g/dl, ESR 50 mm/h, CRP 11.6 mg/dl, and RF 110 U.

Imaging

Detail of the first finger of the right hand. Coronal MR with GE T1-weighted (**a**) and STIR (**b**) sequences shows an erosion of the first metacarpal head. This image is not clearly detectable on conventional radiography (**c**).

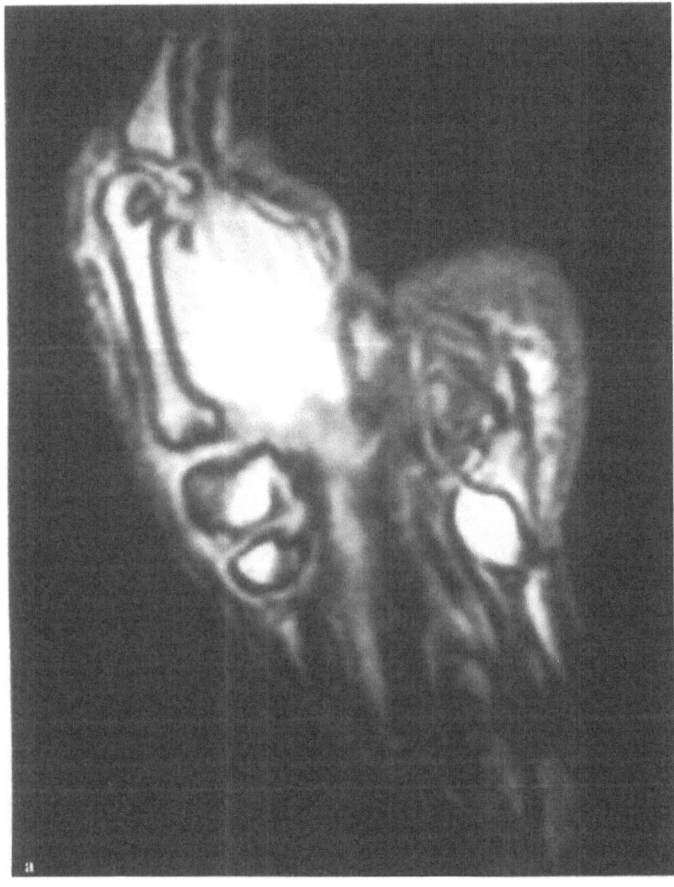

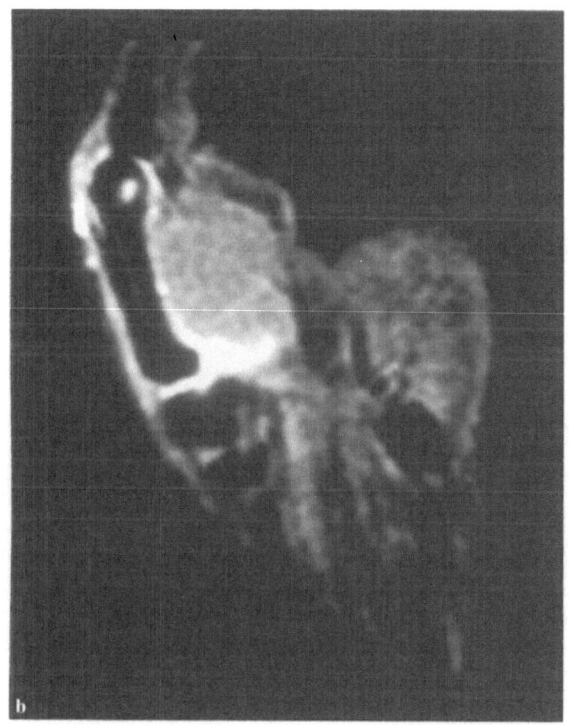

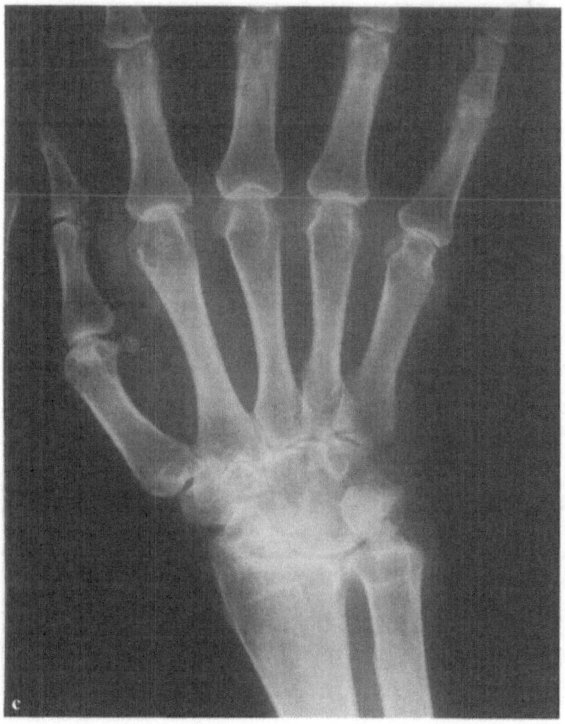

CASE 19

History

This is a 53-year-old woman with a 9-year history of RA which at the time of examination was mild. Hemoglobin was 12.3 g/dl, ESR 6 mm/h, and CRP 5.5 mg/dl.

Imaging

Conventional radiography (**a**) is negative. Coronal GE T1-weighted (**b**) and STIR (**c**) sequences show bone edema with possible early erosions of the distal ulnar epiphysis (*arrow*) and the scaphoid bone (*curved arrow*). MR demonstrates the alteration of the ulnar attachment of the triangular fibrocartilage of the carpus, with associated fluid effusion. Note subchondral bone edema of the scaphoid, depicted as a hyperintense area on the fat-suppressed sequence, and fluid effusion in the midcarpal joints. US scan (**d**) confirms this synovial involvement and power Doppler defines disease activity at the periphery of synovial membrane proliferation.

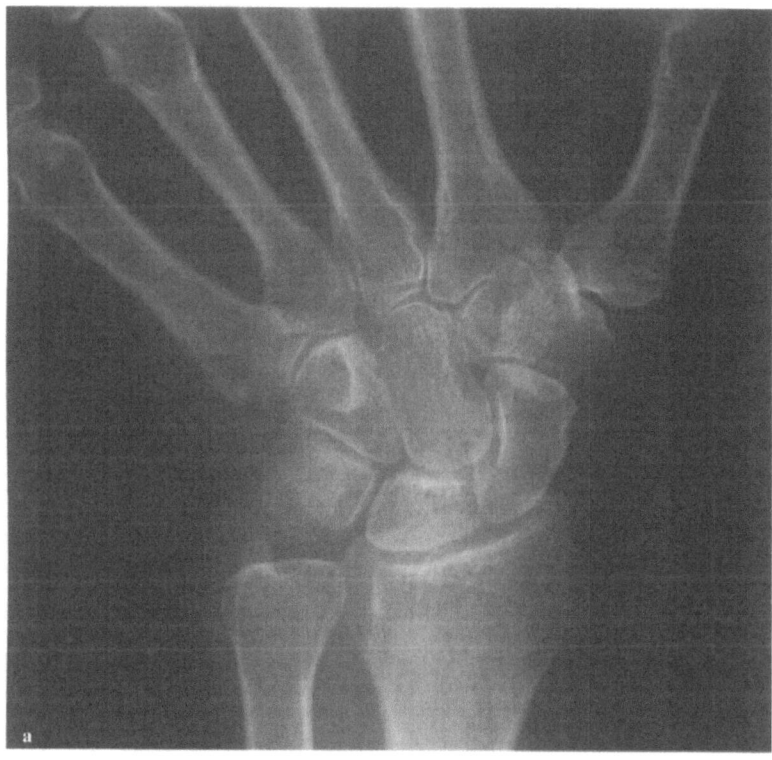

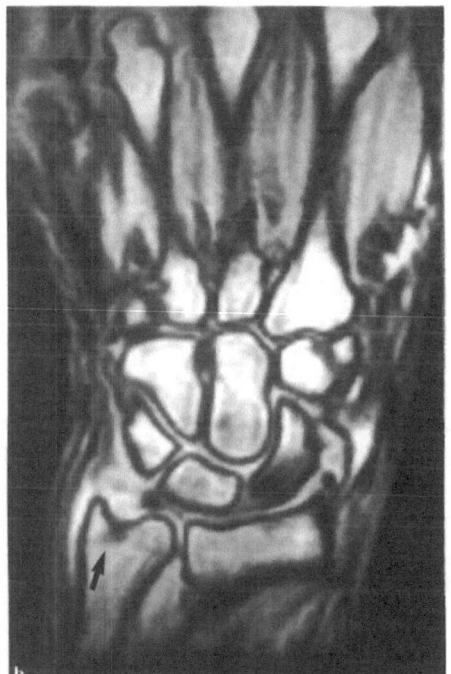

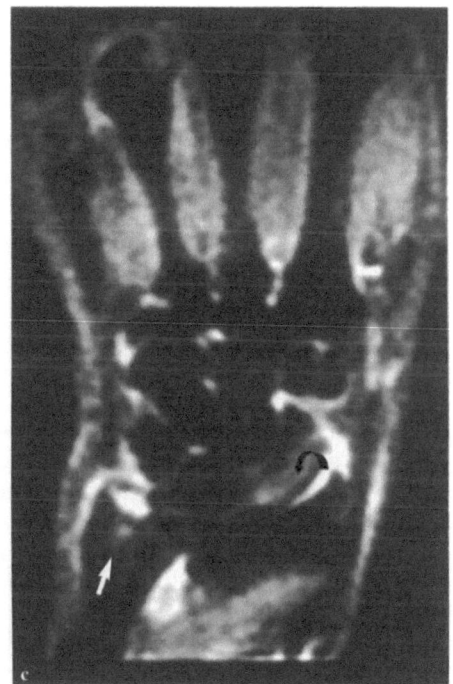

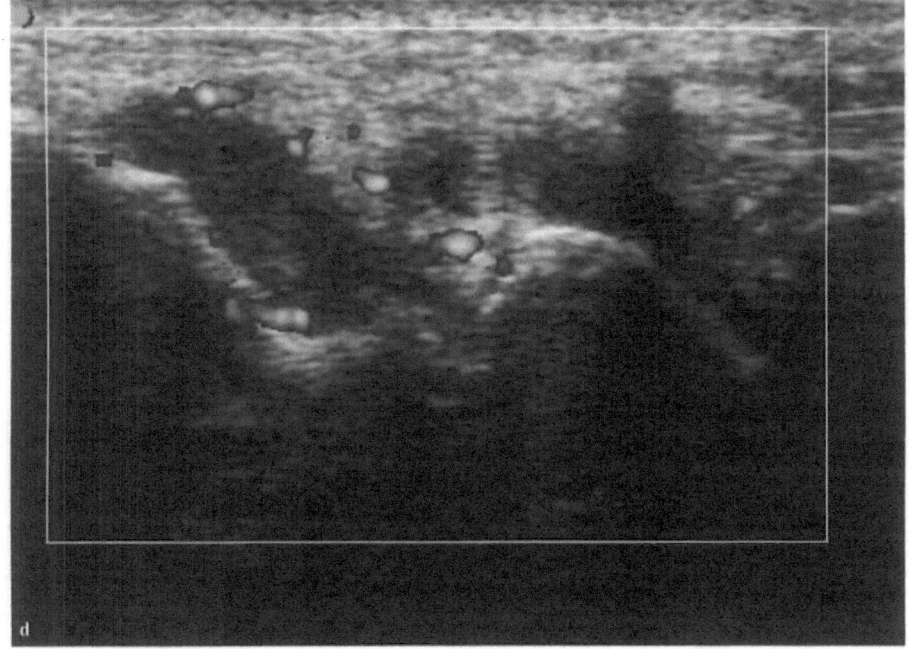

CASE 20

History

This 60-year-old woman had experienced onset of seronegative RA 5 years previously. Disease activity was mild on treatment with gold salts and steroids. Hemoglobin was 12.3 g/dl, ESR 10 mm/h, and CRP 2.8 mg/dl.

Imaging

Axial (**a**) and coronal (**b**) STIR sequences show only an important synovial fluid effusion without bony alterations. In the axial plane, MR demonstrates tenosynovits of the ulnar extensor of carpus (*arrow*) and capsular swelling on the dorsal side of the carpus. US with power Doppler performed on the dorsal aspect of the ulna shows synovial proliferation with only a few vascular spots of small size (**c**).

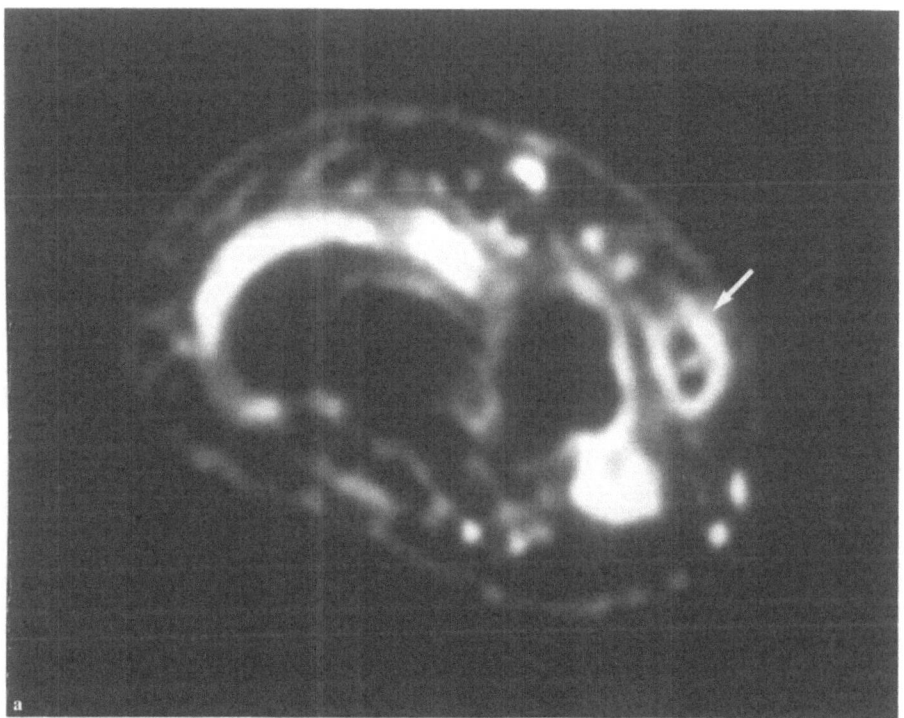

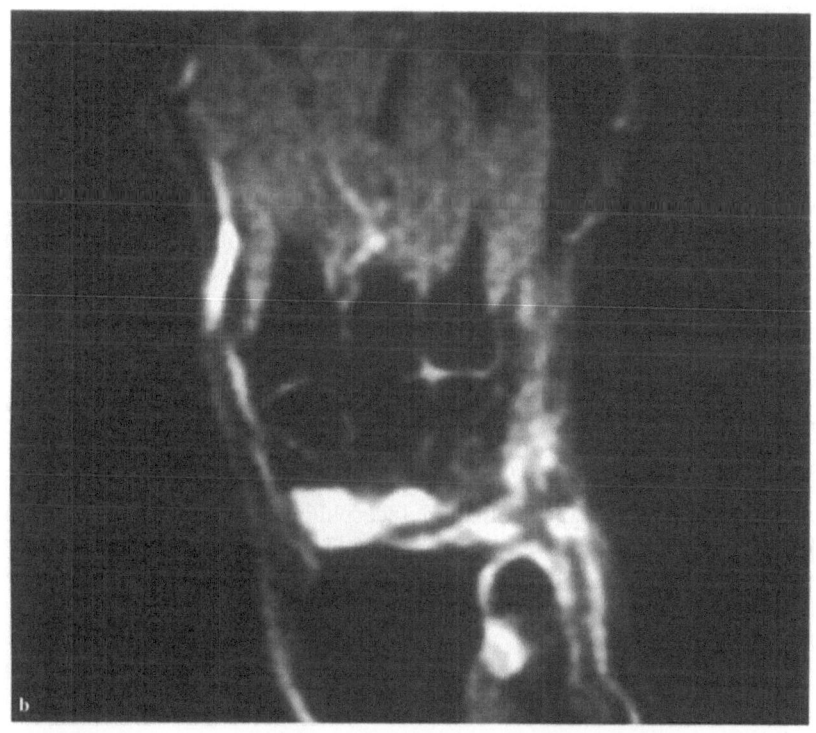

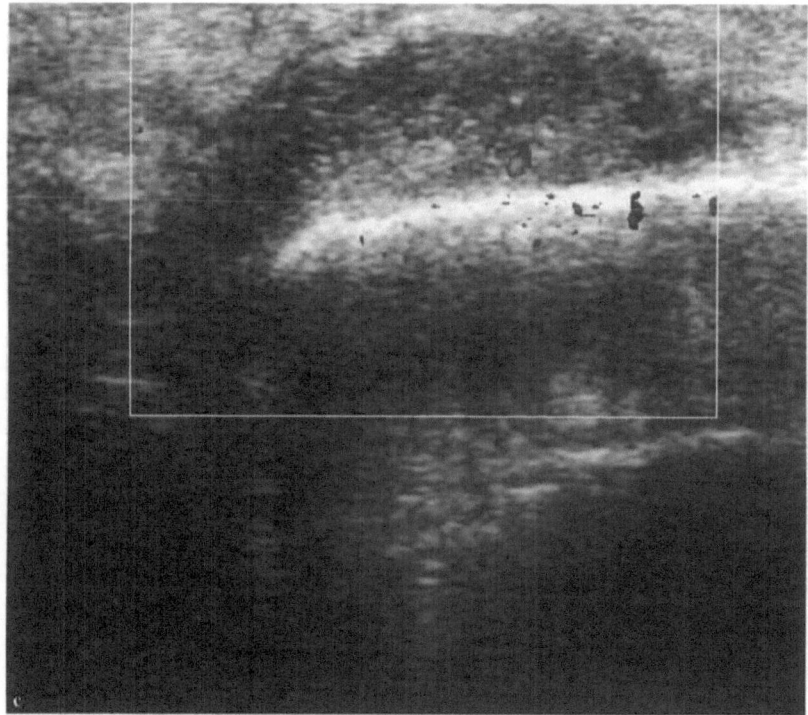

CASE 21

History

This 31-year-old woman had had RA for the past 5 years. She had a period of sustained ACR remission on a combination therapy of steroids, indomethacin, and methotrexate. At this time hemoglobin was 12.3 g/dl, ESR 6 mm/h, and CRP 3 mg/dl.

Imaging

Conventional radiography shows several erosive changes at the base of the second metacarpal and at the third and fourth metacarpal heads (*arrows*). These findings can also be seen in coronal and axial MRI (**b-f**) US shows tenosynovitis of the common extensor tendon (**g**).

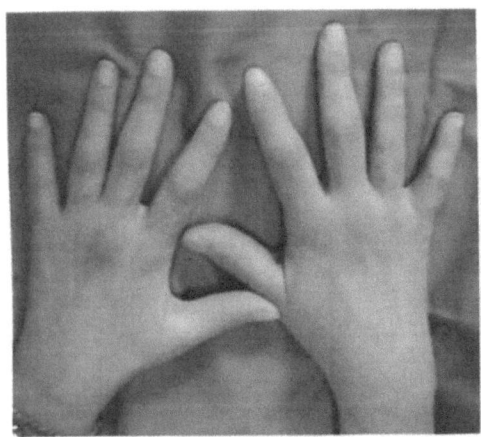

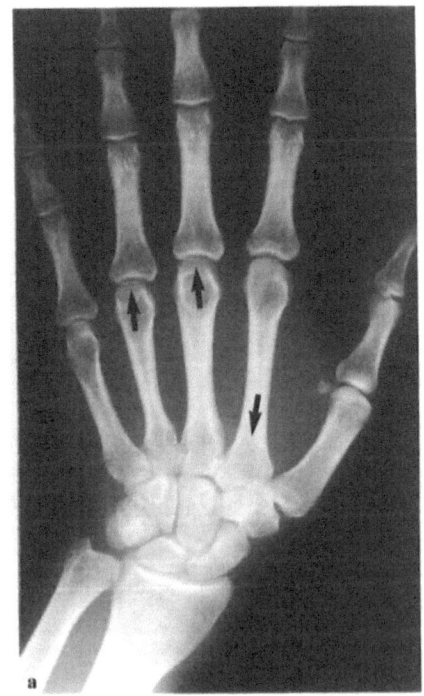

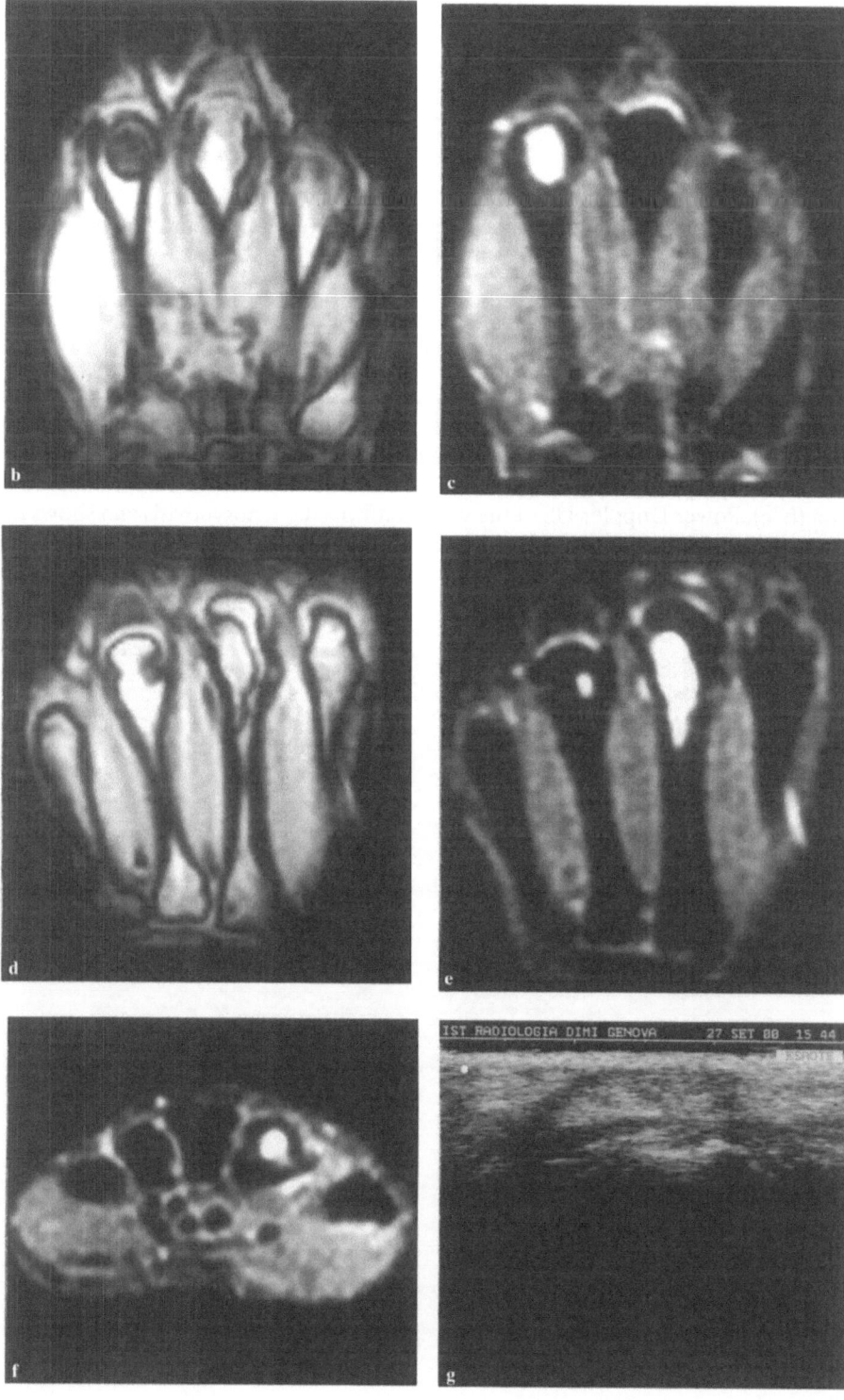

CASE 22

History

A 51-year-old man with a 17-year history of RA had severe joint destruction. At the time of examination, disease activity was relatively low, hemoglobin was 12.8 g/dl, ESR 13 mm/h, and CRP 21.8 mg/dl.

Imaging

A plain film shows carpal fusion and joint space narrowing of the second and third MCP joints, as well as erosions of the ulna (**a**). MRI clearly shows bone lesions, hypertrophic synovial membrane, and tenosynovitis of the extensor carpi radialis tendon (**b, c**). Power Doppler US of the wrist confirms the tenosynovitis and shows intense vascularization of the synovial proliferation (**d**).

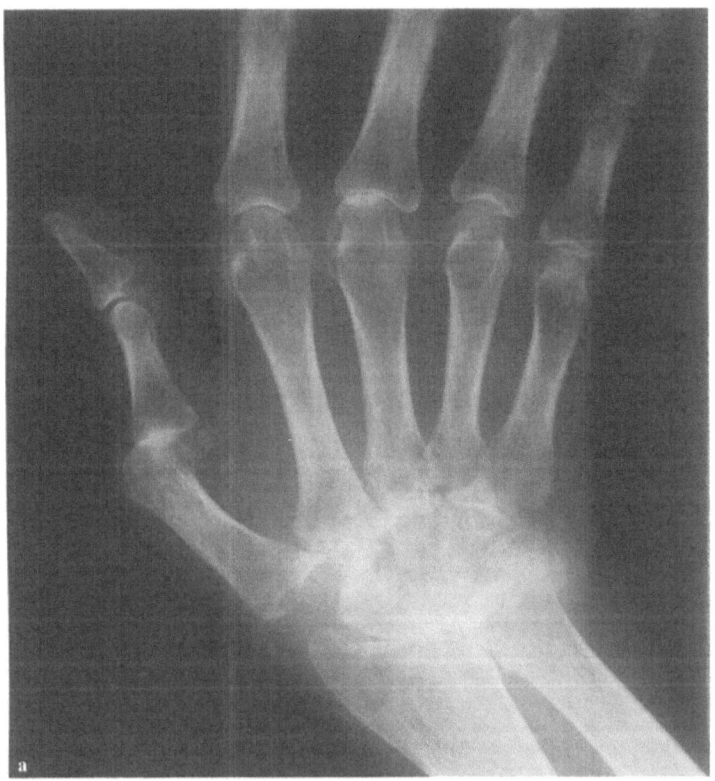

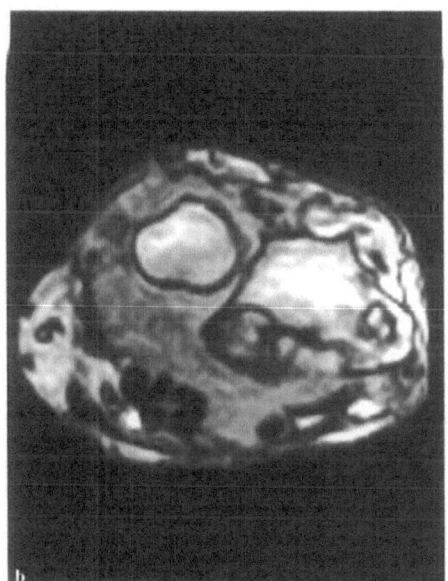
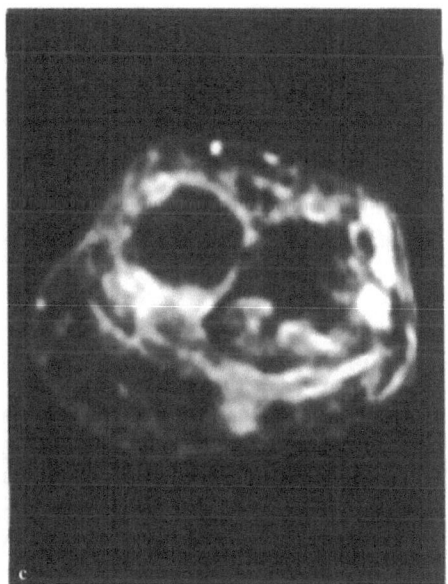

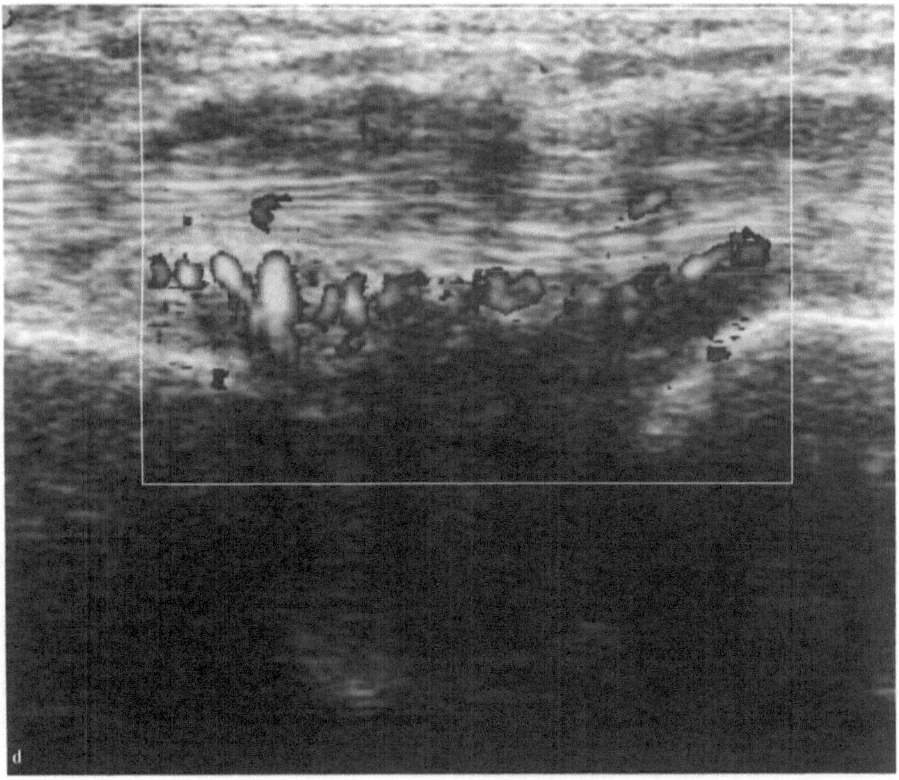

CASE 23

History

This 78-year-old man had suffered from elderly-onset RA for 1 year. Hemoglobin was 13.7 g/dl, ESR 20 mm/h, and CRP 55.2 mg/dl.

Imaging

Radiocarpal joint narrowing and several cystic lesions are seen by conventional radiography (a) of the wrist. Erosions of the capitate, semilunate, and triquetrum are best seen on GE T1-weighted and STIR MR sequences (b, c). Transverse US of the wrist (d) shows change of the structure of the extensor carpi radialis longus, probably due to surrounding inflammation.

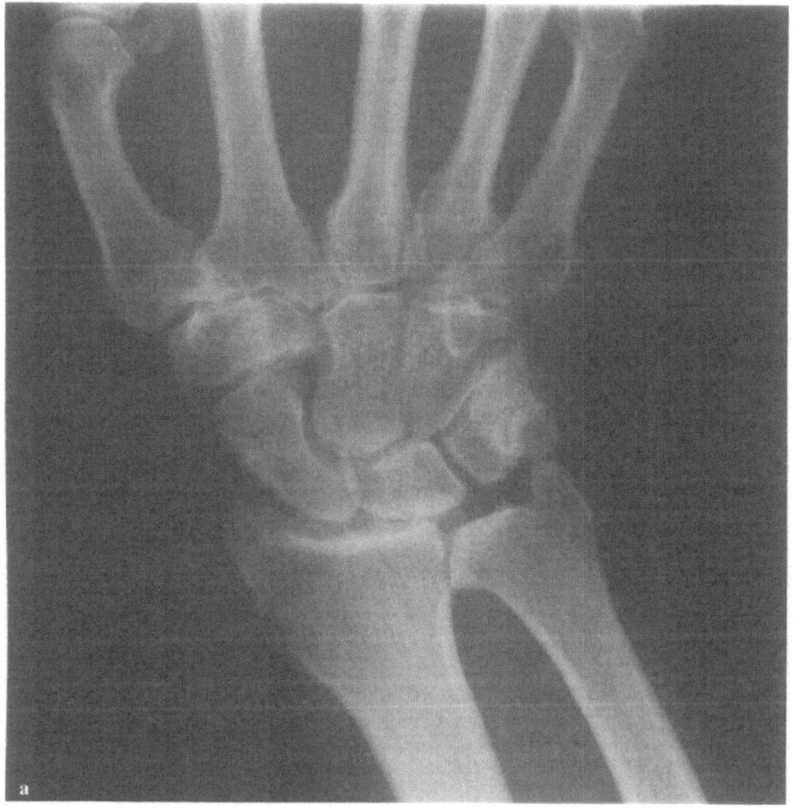

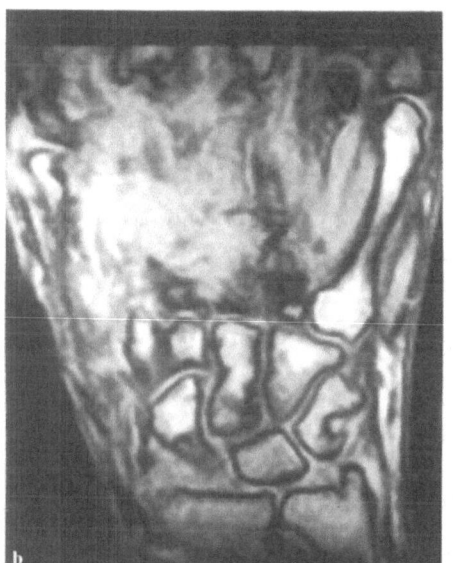

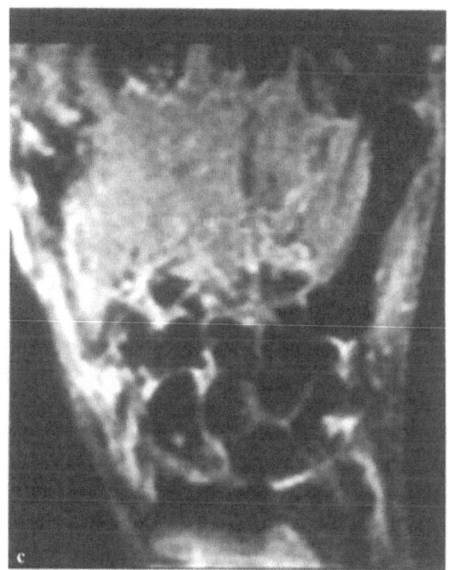

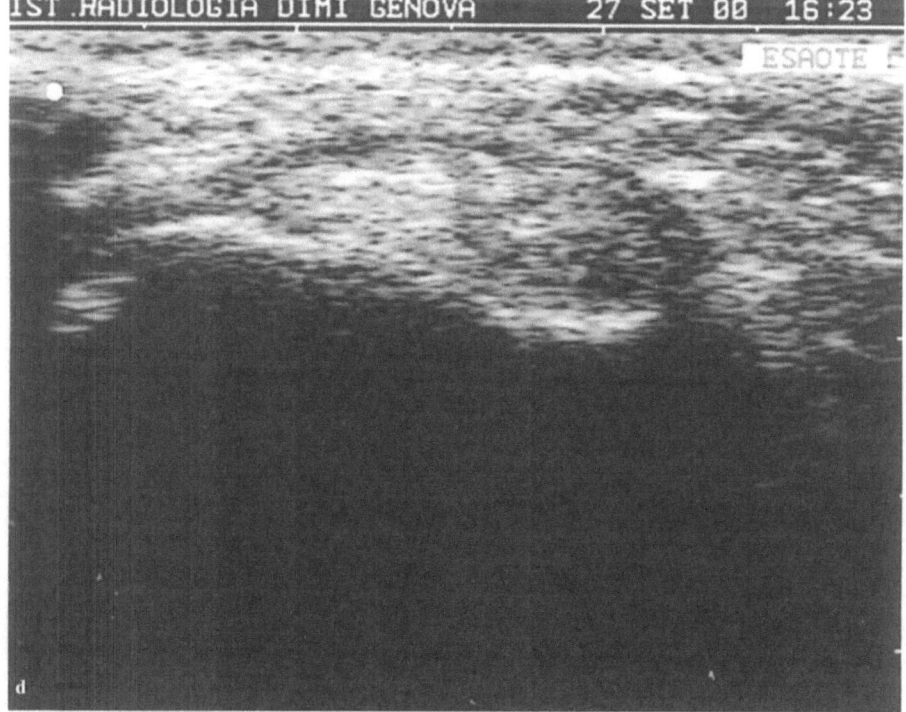

CASE 24

History

This 65-year-old woman had been affected by seropositive RA with nodules for 6 years. She also had concomitant systemic mastocytosis and fibromyalgia which was responsible for at least some of her complaints. Hemoglobin was 10 g/dl, ESR 5 mm/h, and CRP 56 mg/dl.

Imaging

MR shows synovitis of the second MCP joint and the fifth PIP joints (*arrows*). Intense bone edema (*asterisks*), which is hypointense in the GE T1 sequence (**a**) and hyperintense in the STIR sequence (**b**), can be seen in the third and fourth proximal phalanges. Tenosynovitis of the extensor carpi ulnaris is shown in the axial STIR image (**c**). US confirms this last aspect: the synovial sheath has an hypoechoic appearance due to synovial proliferation (*curved arrows*, **d**).

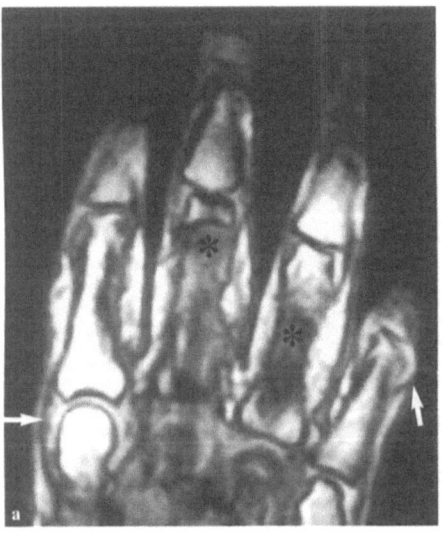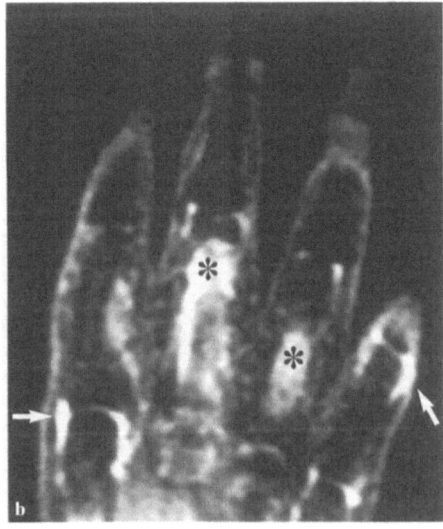

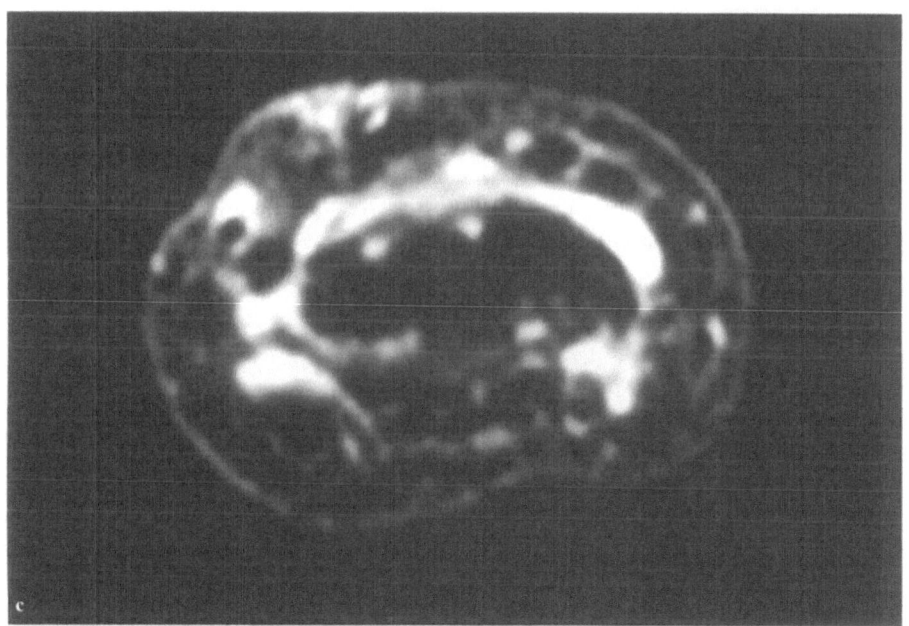

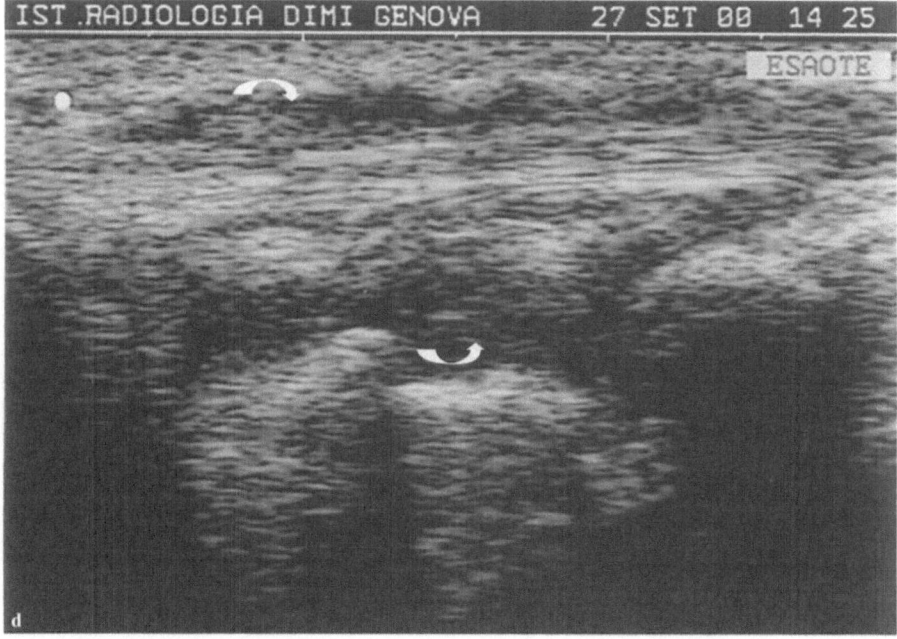

CASE 25

History

This 71-year-old woman had had RA for 5 years. Hemoglobin was 12.3g/dl, ESR 58 mm/h, and CRP 23 mg/dl.

Imaging
In spite of a normal plain film (**a**), MR shows a small erosion at the basis of the first metacarpal bone (*arrow*). This area is hypointense in the T1-weighted sequence (**b**) and hyperintense in the STIR sequence (**c**). The axial sequences show synovial hypertrophy (**d, e**). This area is vascularized, according to the result of Power Doppler analysis (**f**).

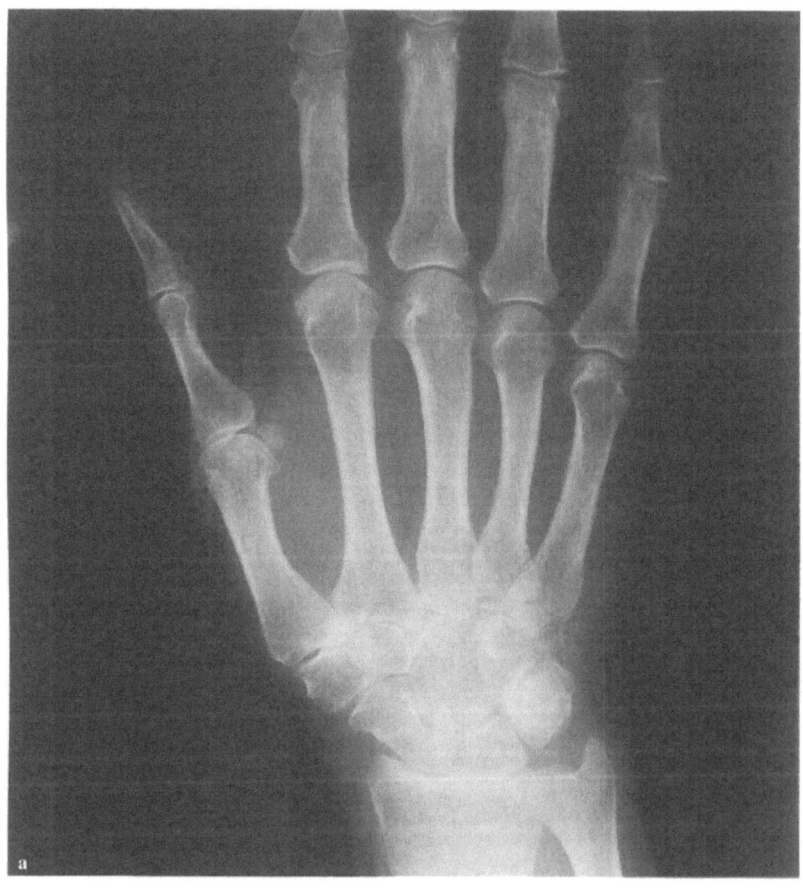

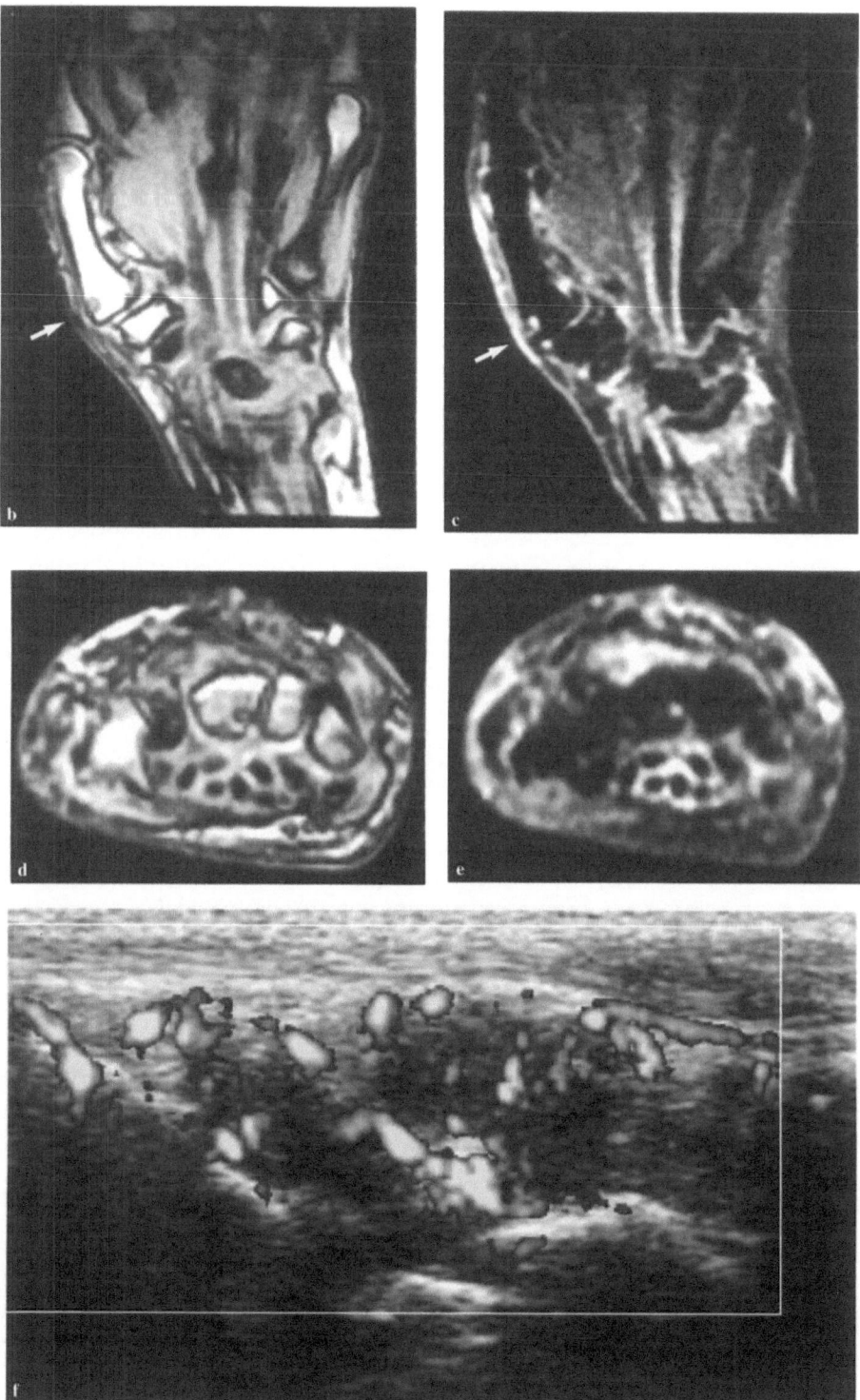

Bibliography

Chapter 1 "History, Epidemiology and Clinical Evaluation of Rheumatoid Arthritis"

Aho K, Heliövaara M, Maatela J, Tuomi T, Palosuo T. Rheumatoid factors antedating clinical rheumatoid arthritis. J Rheumatol 1991; 18:1282-4.

Aho K, Kaipiainen-Seppänen O, Heliövaara M, Klaukka T. Epidemiology of rheumatoid arthritis in Finland. Semin Arthritis Rheum 1998; 27:325-34.

Aho K, Koskenvuo M, Tuominen J, Kaprio J. Occurrence of rheumatoid arthritis in a nationwide series of twins. J Rheumatol 1986; 13:899-902.

Andersson EC, Svendsen P, Svejgaard A, Holmdahl R, Fugger L. A molecule basis for the HLA association in rheumatoid arthritis. Rev Immunogenet 2000; 2:81-7.

Arnett FC, Edworthy SM, Bloch DA, et al. The American Rheumatism Association 1987 revised criteria for the classification of rheumatoid arthritis. Arthritis Rheum 1988; 31:315-24.

Boki KA, Panay GS, Vaughan RW, Drosos AA, Moutsopoulos HM, Lanchbury JS (1992) HLA class II sequence polymorphisms and susceptibility to rheumatoid arthritis in Greeks: the HLA-DRß shared-epitope hyothesis accounts for the disease in only a minority of Greek patients. Arthritis Rheum 35:749-755

Bologna C, Viu P, Jorgensen C, Sany J. Effect of age on the efficacy and tolerance of methotrexate in rheumatoid arthritis. Br J Rheumatol 1996; 35:453-7.

Cimmino MA, Parisi M, Moggiana GL, Mela GS, Accardo S. The prevalence of rheumatoid arthritis in Italy: the Chiavari study. Ann Rheum Dis 1998; 57:315-8.

Cimmino MA. Geographical differences in the prevalence and severity of rheumatoid arthritis in Europe. CPD Bull Rheumatol Arthritis 1999; 1:28-34.

Del Puente A, Knowler WC, Pettitt DJ, Bennett PH. The incidence of rheumatoid arthritis is predicted by rheumatoid factor titer in a longitudinal population study. Arthritis Rheum 1988; 31:1239-45.

Dequeker J. Rheumatic diseases in visual arts. General review. In: Appelboom T (ed.) Art, history and antiquity of rheumatic diseases. Elsevier, Brussels; 1987:84.

Dugowson CE, Koepsell TD, Voigt LF, Bley L, Nelson JL, Daling JR. Rheumatoid arthritis in women: incidence rates in a group health cooperative, Seattle, Washington 1987-1989. Arthritis Rheum 1991; 34:1502-7.

Ferraccioli GF, Salaffi F, Troise-Rioda W, Bartoli E. The chronic arthritis systemic index (CASI). Clin Exp Rheumatol 1994; 12:241-7.

Garrod AB. The nature and treatment of gout and rheumatoid gout. London, Walton and Maberley; 1859.

Hameed K, Gibson T, Kadir M, Sultana S, Fatima Z, Syed A. The prevalence of rheumatoid arthritis in affluent and poor urban communities of Pakistan. Br J Rheumatol 1995; 34:252-6.

Harris ED Jr. Rheumatoid arthritis: pathophysiology and implications for therapy. N Engl J Med 1990; 322:1277-89.

Imanaka T, Shichikawa K, Inoue K, et al. Increase in age at onset of rheumatoid arthritis in Japan over a 30 year period. Ann Rheum Dis 1997; 56:313-6.

Kaipiainen-Seppanen O, Aho K, Nikkarinen M. Regional differences in the incidence of rheumatoid arthritis in Finland in 1995. Ann Rheum Dis 2001; 60:128-32.

Kaltenhauser S, Wagner U, Schuster E, et al. Immunogenetic markers and seropositivity predict radiological progression in early rheumatoid arthritis independent of disease activity. J Rheumatol 2001; 28:735-44.

Kanik KS, Wilder RL. Hormonal alterations in rheumatoid arthritis, including the effects of pregnancy. Rheum Dis Clin North Am. 2000; 26:805-23.

Kurumbail RG, Stevens AM, Gierse JK, et al. Structural basis for selective inhibition of cyclooxygenase-2 by anti-inflammatory agents. Nature 1996; 384:644-8.

Laan RF, van Riel PL, van De Putte LB. Leflunomide and methotrexate. Curr Opin Rheumatol 2001; 13:159-63.

Lipsky PE, van der Heijde DM, St Clair EW, Furst DE, Breedveld FC, Kalden JR, Smolen JS, Weisman M, Emery P, Feldmann M, Harriman GR, Maini RN. Infliximab and methotrexate in the treatment of rheumatoid arthritis. Anti-Tumor Necrosis Factor Trial in Rheumatoid Arthritis with Concomitant Therapy Study Group. N Engl J Med 2000; 343:1594-602.

O'Dell JR, Haire CE, Erikson N, et al. Treatment of rheumatoid arthritis with methotrexate alone, sulfasalazine and hydroxychloroquine, or a combination of all three medications. N Engl J Med 1996; 334:1287-91.

Pasero G, Priolo P, Marubini E, et al. Slow progression of joint damage in early rheumatoid arthritis treated with cyclosporin A. Arthritis Rheum 1996; 39:1006-15.

Rothschild BM, Woods RJ, Rothschild C, Sebes JI. Geographic distribution of rheumatoid arthritis in ancient North America: implications for pathogenesis. Semin Arthritis Rheum 1992; 22:181-7.

Salvarani C, Macchioni PL, Mantovani M, et al. HLA-DRB1 alleles associated with rheumatoid arthritis in northern Italy: correlation with disease severity. Br J Rheumatol 1998; 37:165-9.

Seriolo B, Accardo S, Fasciolo D, Bertolini S, Cutolo M. Lipoproteins, anticardiolipin antibodies and thrombotic events in rheumatoid arthritis. Clin Exp Rheumatol 1996; 14:593-9.

Silman AJ, Davies P, Currey HLF, Evans SJW. Is rheumatoid arthritis becoming less severe? J Chron Dis 1983; 36:891-7.

Silman AJ, Ollier WO, Holligan S, Birrel F, Adebajo A, Asuzu MC, Thomson W, Pepper L. Absence of rheumatoid arthritis in a rural Nigerian population. J Rheumatol 1993; 20:618-22.

Symmons DPM, Barrett EM, Bankhead CR, Scott DGI, Silman AJ. The occurrence of rheumatoid arthritis in the United Kingdom: results from the Norfolk Arthritis Register. Br J Rheumatol 1994; 33:735-9.

Van der Heijde DMFM, van Riel PLCM, van Rijswijk MH, et al. Influence of prognostic features on the final outcome in rheumatoid arthritis: a review of the literature. Semin Arthritis Rheum 1988; 17:284-92.

Van der Hejde DMFM, van't Hof MA, van Riel PLCM, et al. Judging disease activity in clinical practice in rheumatoid arthritis: first step in the development of a disease activity score. Ann Rheum Dis 1990; 49:919-20.

Vittecoq O, Jouen-Beades F, Krzanowska K, et al. Rheumatoid factors, anti-filaggrin antibodies and low in vitro interleukin-2 and interferon-gamma production are useful immunological markers for early diagnosis of community cases of rheumatoid arthritis. A preliminary study. Joint Bone Spine. 2001; 68:144-53.

Walsh DA, Pearson CI. Angiogenesis in the pathogenesis of inflammatory joint and lung diseases. Arthritis Res. 2001; 3:147-53.

Wolfe F, Mitchell DM, Sibley JT, et al. The mortality of rheumatoid arthritis. Arthritis Rheum 1994; 37:481-94.

Chapter 2 "Conventional Radiography"

Arnett FC, Edworthy SM, Bloch DA. The American Rheumatism Association 1987 revised criteria for the classification of rheumatoid arthritis. Arthritis Rheum. 1988; 31:315-324.

Backhaus M, Kamradt T, Sandrock D, Loreck D, Fritz J, Wolf KJ, Raber H, Hamm B, Burmester GR, Bollow M. Arthritis of the finger joints: a comprehensive approach comparing conventional radiography, scintigraphy, ultrasound and CE magnetic resonance imaging. Arthritis Rheum. 1999 Jun; 42 (6):1232-1245.

Berens DL, Lin RK (editors) (1969) Roentgen Diagnosis of Rheumatoid Arthritis Springfield.

Brahme OK, Gundiy CR, Resnick D. Advanced imaging of the wrist. Radiol. Clin. North Am. 1990; 28 (2):307-320.

Brook A, Corbett M Radiographic changes in early rheumatoid disease. Ann. Rheum. Dis. 1977; 36:71-73.

Cammisa M et al. (1988) Le malattie reumatiche, inquadramento e diagnosi radiologica. Ciba - Geigy, Origgio (VA).

Gardner DL (1978) Pathology of rheumatoid arthritis. Churchill Livingstone, Edinburgh.

Ghadially FN (1983) Fine structure of synovial joints. Butterworths, London.

Grassi W, De Angelis R, Lamanna G, Cervini C. The clnical features of rheumaotid arthritis. Eur J Radiol 1998; 27:18-24.

Jaffe HL (1972) Metabolic, degenerative and inflammatory disease of bones and joints. Lea and Febiger, Philadelphia.

Kaarela K, Kautiainen H Continuos progression of radiological destruction in sieropositive rheumatoid arthritis. J Rheumatol 1997 Jul; 24 (7):1285-1287.

Kaye JJ, Nance EP, Callahan LF. Observer variation in quantitative assessment of rheumatoid arthritis. Part II. A simplified scoring system. Invest Radiol 1987; 22:41-46.

Larsen A. How to apply Larsen score in evaluating radiographs of rheumatoid arthritis in long term studies. J Rheumatol 1995; 22:1975.

Martel W. The pattern of rheumatoid arthritis in the hand and wrist. Radiol Clin North Am 1964; 2:221.

Resnick D (1995) Diagnosis of bones and joints disorders. Saunders, Philadelphia.

Resnick D. Rheumatoid arthritis of the wrist. The compartmental approach. Med Radiogr Photogr 1976; 52:50.

Sharp JT, Litsky MD, Collins LC et al. Methods of scoring the progression of radiologic changes in rheumatoid arthritis: correlation of radiologic and laboratory abnormalities. Arthritis Rheum 1971; 14:706-720.

Trentham DE, Masi AT. Carpo-metacarpal ratio. A new quantitative measure of radiologic progression of wrist involvement in rheumatoid arthritis. Arthritis Rheum 1976; 19:939.

Chapter 2 "Ultrasonography"

Aisen AM, Mc Cune WJ, MacGuire A, et al Sonographic evaluation of the cartilage of the knee. Radiology, 1984; 153:781.

Beecker HK (1959) Measurement of Subjective Responses. New York, Oxford University Press.

Buchberger W, Jadmaier W, Birbamer G, et al. Carpal tunnel syndrome: diagnosis with high resolution sonography. AJR 1992; 159:793-798.

Chen P, Maklad N, Redwine M, Zelitt D Dynamic high resolution sonography of the carpal tunnel. AJR 1997; 168:533-537.

Chiou HJ, Chang CY, Chou YH, et al Triangular fibrocartilage of the wrist: Presentation on high resolution ultrasonography. J Ultrasound Med 1998; 17:41-48.

Giovagnorio F, Andreoli C, De Cicco ML Ultrasonographic evaluation of De Quervaine disease. J Ultrasound Med 1997 16:685-689.

Koski JM, Anttila P, Hamalainen M, et al Hip joint ultrasonography: correlation with intra-articular effusion and synovitis. Br J Rheum 1990; 29, 189.

Marnix Van Holsbeeck, J Introcaso (1991): Musculoskeletal ultrasound, Mosby Year Book.

Martino F, Monetti G (1993) Semeiotica ecografica delle malattie reumatiche, Piccin.

Reinhardt M, Fritzsch T. Caratteristiche e applicazioni: attualità e prospettive. Radiol Med 1998; 95 (Suppl. 1 al N. 5): 1-5.

Richardson ML, Selby B, Montana MA, et al Ultrasonography of the knee. Radiol Clin North Am 1988; 26(1):63.

Ropes MW, Bennett GA, Cobb S et al Revision of the diagnostic criteria of rheumatoid arthritis. Ann Rheum Dis 1959; 18:49.

Rubin JM, Bude RO, Carson PL, Bree RL, Adler RS. Power Doppler: a potentially useful alternative to mean-frequency based color Doppler sonography. Radiology 1994; 190: 853-856.

Silvestri E, Martinoli C, Derchi LE, et al Echotexture of peripheral nerves: correlation between US and histologic findings and criteria to differentiate tendons. Radiology 1995; 197:291-296.

Silvestri E, Martinoli C, Onetto, F, Neumaier CE, Cimmino MA, Derchi LE. Valutazione dell'artrite reumatoide del ginocchio con color Doppler. Radiol Med 1994; 88:364-367.

Van Holsbeeck M, Van Holsbeeck K, Gevers G, et al Staging and follow up of Reumathoid Arthritis of the knee. Comparison of sonography, thermography, and clinical assessment. J Ultrasound Med 1988, 7: 561-566.

Chapter 2 "Magnetic Resonance"

Arner M, Jonsson K, Aspenberg P. Complete palmar dislocation of the lunate in rheumatoid arthritis. Avascularity without avascular changes. J Hand Surg [Br] 1996; 21:384-387.

Beltran J, Caudill JC, Herman LH, Kantor SM, Hudson PN, Noto AM, et al. Rheumatoid arthritis: MR manifestations. Radiology 1987; 165:153-7.

Bjorkengren AG, Geborek P, Rydholm U, Holtås S, Petterson H. MR imaging of the knee in acute rheumatoid arthritis: synovial uptake of gadolinium-DOTA. Am J Roentgenol 1990; 155:329-32.

Brahme SK, Gundry CR, Resnick D. Advanced imaging of the wrist. Radiol Clin North Am 1990; 28:307-320.

Brahme SK, Resnick D. Magnetic resonance imaging of the wrist. Rheum Dis Clin North Am 1991; 17:721-739.

Cimmino MA, Garlaschi G, Bountis C, Silvestri E, Delucchi S, Frisone G, et al. Reproducibility of magnetic resonance (MR) readings of erosions in the rheumatoid wrist. Arthritis Rheum 1998; 41(Abstract): S51.

Corvetta A, Giovagnoni A, Baldelli S, Ercolani P, Pomponio G, Luchetti MM, et al. MR imaging of rheumatoid hand lesions: comparison with conventional radiology in 31 patients. Clin Exp Rheumatol 1992; 10:217-222.

Delfaut EM, Beltran J, Johnson G, Rousseau J, Marchandise X, Cotten A. Fat suppression in MR imaging: techniques and pitfalls. Radiographics 1999; 19:372-82.

Dooley MA, Messina JP, Gilkeson GS, Spritzer CE, Pisetsky DS. MRI features in early rheumatoid arthritis correlation with clinical and immunological response to NSAID therapy. Arthritis Rheum 1991; 34 (Abstract): S63

Dooley MA, Pisetsky DS, Scarlett EL, Gilkeson GS, Collins AJ, Spritzer CE. Longitudinal MRI studies in early RA: correlation with clinical and radiographic disease activity. Arthritis Rheum 1992; 35 (Abstract): S196

Foley-Nolan D, Stack JP, Ryan M, Redmond U, Barry C, Ennis J, et al. Magnetic resonance imaging in the assessment of rheumatoid arthritis – a comparison with plain film radiographs. Br J Rheumatol 1991; 30:101-106.

Franklin PD, Lemon RA, Barden HS. Accuracy of imaging the menisci on an in-office, dedicated magnetic resonance imaging extremity system. Am J Sports Med 1997; 25:382-7.

Gilkenson G, Polisson R, Sinclair HD, Vogler J, Rice J, Caldwell D, et al.. Early detection of carpal erosions in patients with rheumatoid arthritis: a pilot study of magnetic resonance imaging. J Rheumatol 1988; 15:1361-6.

Giovagnoni A, Baldelli S, Ercolani P, Misericordia M, Corvetta A, Lucchetti MM, et al. Magnetic resonance of the rheumatoid hand. Radiol Med (Torino) 1991; 81:396-403.

Giovagnoni A, Ercolani P, Soccetti A, Misericordia M, De Nigris E. Magnetic resonance imaging of carpal tunnel syndrome. Radiol Med 1991; 82:35-39.

Gubler FM, Algra PR, Maas M, Dijkstra PF, Falke TH. Gadolinium-DTPA enhanced magnetic resonance imaging of bone cysts in patients with rheumatoid arthritis. Ann Rheum Dis 1993; 520:716-719.

Gubler FM, Maas M, Dijkstra PF, de Jongh HR. Cystic rheumatoid arthritis: description of a nonerosive form. Radiology 1990; 177:829-34.

Hug C, Huber I, Terrier F, Häuselmann HJ, Aue W, Vock P, et al. Detection of flexor tenosynovitis by magnetic resonance imaging: its relationship to diurnal variation of symptoms. J Rheumatol 1991; 18:1055-59.

Jevtic V, Watt I, Rozman B, Kos-Golja M, Demsar F, Jath O. Use of contrast-enhanced MRI in the assessment of therapeutic response to a disease-modifying antirheumatic drug. Case study. Br J Rheum 1995; 34:956-959.

Jevtic V, Watt I, Rozman B, Kos-Golja M, Rupenovic S, Logar D, et al. Precontrast and postcontrast (Gd-DTPA) magnetic resonance imaging of hand joints in patients with rheumatoid arthritis. Clin Radiol 1993; 48:176-181.

Jevtic V, Watt I, Rozman B, Kos-Goljia M, Praprotnik S, Logar D, et al. Contrast enhanced Gd-DTPA magnetic resonance imaging in evaluation of rheumatoid arthritis during a clinical trial with DMARDs. A prospective two-year follow-up study on hand joints in 31 patients. Clin Exp Rheum 1997; 15:151-156.

Jorgensen C, Cyteval C, Anaya JM, Baron MP, Lamarque JL, Sany J. Sensitivity of magnetic resonance imaging of the wrist in very early rheumatoid arthritis. Clin Exp Rheumatol 1993; 11:163-168.

Kersting-Sommerhoff B, Hof N, Lenz M, Gerhardt P. MRI of peripheral joints with a low-field dedicated system: a reliable and cost-effective alternative to high-field units? Eur Radiol 1996; 6:561-5.

König H, Lucas D, Meissner R. The wrist: a preliminary report on high-resolution MR imaging. Radiology 1986; 160:463-467.

Krahe T, Landwehr P, Stolzenburg T, Richthammer A, Schindler R, Lackner K. Magnetic resonance tomography (MRT) of the hand in chronic polyarthritis. Rofo Fortschr Geb Rontgenstr Neuen Bildgeb Verfahr 1990; 152:206-213.

Lee J, Lee SK, Suh JS, Yoon M, Song JH, Lee CH. Magnetic resonance imaging of the wrist in defining remission of rheumatoid arthritis. J Rheumatol 1997; 24:1303-1308.

Link TM, Bongertz GM, Böger K, Heinke Daldrup, Smitz-Linneweber B, Peters PE. Einsatz von Gadoteridol in der MR-Diagnostik rheumatoider Gelenkveränderungen. Radiologe 1996; 36:141-147.

Mc Queen FM, Stewart N, Crabbe J, Robinson E, Yeoman S, Tan PLJ, et al. Magnetic resonance imaging of the wrist in early rheumatoid arthritis reveals a high prevalence of erosions at four months after symptom onset. Ann Rheum Dis 1998; 57:350-356.

McGonagle D, Gibbon W, Green M, Proudmann S, O'Connor P, Emery P. A longitudinal MR study of the relationship between synovitis, bone oedema and bone erosion in early rheumatoid arthritis. Br J Rheumatol 1998, 37 (Abstract): 105.

McGonagle D, Green MJ, Proudman S, Richardson C, Veale D, O'Connor P, et al. The majority of patients with rheumatoid arthritis have erosive disease at presentation when MRI of the dominant hand is employed. Br J Rheumatol 1997; 36 (Suppl 1) (Abstract): 121.

Mesgarzadeh M, Schneck CD, Bonakdarpour A, Mitra A, Conaway D. Carpal tunnel: MR imaging. Part II. Carpal tunnel syndrome. Radiology 1989; 171:749-754.

Meske S, Friedburg H, Hennig J, Reinbold W, Stappert K, Schumichen C. Rheumatoid arthritis lesions of the wrist examined by rapid gradient-echo magnetic resonance imaging. Scand J Rheumatol 1990; 19:235-238.

Meske S, Stappert K, Friedburg H, Mundinger A. Attempt at staging articular changes in rheumatoid arthritis using magnetic resonance tomography exemplified by the wrist joint. Z Rheumatol 1990; 49:294-297.

Nägele M, Kunze V, Koch W, Brüning R, Seelos K, Ströhmann I, et al. Rheumatoid arthritis of the wrist. Dynamic Gd-DTPA enhanced MRT. Rofo Fortschr Geb Rontgenstr Neuen Bildgeb Verfahr 1993; 158:141-146.

Nakahara N, Uetani M, Hayashi K, Kawahara Y, Matsumoto T, Oda J. Gadolinium-enhanced MR imaging of the wrist in rheumatoid arthritis: value of fat suppression pulse sequences. Skeletal Radiol 1996; 25:639-647.

Østergaard M, Gideon P, Sorensen K, Hansen M, Stoltenberg M, Henriksen O, et al. Scoring of synovial membrane hypertrophy and bone erosions by MR imaging in clinically active and inactive rheumatoid arthritis of the wrist. Scand J Rheumatol 1995; 24:212-218.

Østergaard M, Hansen M, Stoltenberg M, Lorenzen I. Quantitative assessment of the synovial membrane in the rheumatoid wrist: an easily obtained MRI score reflects the synovial volume. Br J Rheumatol 1996; 35:965-971.

Østergaard M. Different approaches to synovial membrane volume determination by magnetic resonance imaging: manual versus automated segmentation. Br J Rheumatol 1997; 36:1166-77.

Palmer WE, Rosenthal DI, Schoenberg OI, Fischman AJ, Simon LS, Rubin RH, et al. Quantification of inflammation in the wrist with gadolinium-enhanced MR imaging and PET with 2-[F-18]-fluoro-2-deoxy-D-glucose. Radiology 1995; 196:647-655.

Pierre-Jerome C, Bekkelund SI, Husby G, Mellgren SI, Torbergsen T. Bilateral fast MR imaging of the rheumatoid wrist. Clin Rheumatol 1996; 15:42-46.

Pierre-Jerome C, Bekkelund SI, Mellgren SI, Torbergsen T, Husby G, Nordstrom R. The rheumatoid wrist: bilateral MR analysis of the distribution of rheumatoid lesions in axial plane in a female population. Clin Rheumatol 1997; 16:80-86.

Polisson RP, Schoenberg OI, Fischman A, Rubin R, Simon LS, Rosenthal D, et al. Use of magnetic resonance imaging and positron emission tomography in the assessment of synovial volume and glucose metabolism in patients with rheumatoid arthritis. Arthritis Rheum 1995; 38:819-825.

Reiser MF, Bongartz GP, Erlemann R, Schneider M, Pauly T, Sittek H, et al. Gadolinium-DTPA in rheumatoid arthritis and related disease: first results with dynamic resonance imaging. Skeletal Radiol 1989; 18:591-7.

Reiser MF, Schneider M, Sittek H, Bongartz GP. Stellenwert der Magnetresonanz-tomographie (MTR) bei entzüntlich-rheumatischen Erkrankungen. Z Rheumatol 1990; 49:61-9.

Rominger MB, Bernreuter WK, Kenney PJ, Morgan SL, Blackburn WD, Alarcon GS. MR Imaging of the hands in early rheumatoid arthritis: preliminary results. Radiographics 1993; 13:37-46.

Rubens DJ, Blebea JS, Totterman SM, Hooper MM. Rheumatoid arthritis: evaluation of wrist extensor tendons with clinical examination versus MR imaging - a preliminary report. Radiology 1993; 187:831-838.

Sugimoto H, Takeda A, Kano S. Assessment of disease activity in rheumatoid arthritis using magnetic resonance imaging: quantification of pannus volume in the hands. Br J Rheumatol 1998; 37:854-861.

Sugimoto H, Takeda A, Masuyama J, Furuse M. Early-stage rheumatoid arthritis: diagnostic accuracy of MR imaging. Radiology 1996; 198:185-192.

Tonolli-Serabian I, Poet JL, Dufour M, Carasset S, Mattei JP, Roux H. Magnetic resonance imaging of the wrist in rheumatoid arthritis: comparison with other inflammatory joint diseases and control subjects. Clin Rheumatol 1996; 15:137-142.

Winalski CS, Palmer WE, Rosenthal DI, Weissman BN. Magnetic resonance imaging of rheumatoid arthritis. Radiol Clin North Am 1996; 34:243-58.

Yanagawa A, Takano K, Nishioka K, Shimada J, Mizushima Y, Ashida H. Clinical staging and gadolinium-DTPA enhanced images of the wrist in rheumatoid arthritis. J Rheumatol 1993; 20:781-784.